Yoga-sūtra of Patañjali

Yoga-sūtra of Patañjali

by

Saugata Bhaduri

D.K.Printworld(P)Ltd.
NEW DELHI - 110 015

Cataloging in Publication Data — DK

Bhaduri, Saugata, 1972 –
Yoga-sūtra of Patañjali.
Includes index.

1. Patañjali. Yogasūtra. 2. Yoga. 3. Philosophy, Hindu. I. Patañjali. Yogasūtra. English & Sanskrit. 2000. II. Title.

ISBN 81-246-0157-7

First Published in India in 2000

Second impression in 2006

Published and printed by:
D.K. Printworld (P) Ltd.
Regd. office : *'Sri Kunj'*, F-52, Bali Nagar
New Delhi - 110 015
Phones : (011) 545-3975, 546-6019; *Fax* : (011) 546-5926
E-mail: dkprint@4mis.com

Foreword

UNDER the guidance of Prof. Kapil Kapoor at the Centre of Linguistics and English, JNU, in 1995, a group of scholars was assigned to take up the primary text of any one of the nine schools of classical Indian philosophy and translate it keeping in mind the needs of Indian students, who are familiar with many of the concepts dealt with in these texts through their mother tongues but not comfortable enough with Sanskrit grammar to peruse the same in the original. The enthusiasm we showed for this project made Prof. Kapoor informally constitute a group called the Śāstra Group, whose avowed purpose was to fulfil in the years to come the onerous task that we wilfully took upon our young, weak and rather too ambitious shoulders. It is quite heartening to present this book in its current form and relive some of the enthusiasm we shared in those days of the past when not the worry about how to keep our hearths burning but the burning desire to do something meaningful with our rich cultural past fuelled us on.

Nostalgia apart, what would be worthwhile to mention in this 'Foreword' is how this translation is different from the numerous English versions of Patañjali's *Yoga-sūtra* that are already available. Three features mark these existing translations and make them unsuitable for the intended reader that this volume presupposes — the Indian student. First, all these translations try to find one-word English equivalents for virtually untranslatable Sanskrit technical terms, leading to extremely inadequate renderings of pregnant words. This work, on the contrary, retains many Sanskrit terms in the translation, assuming that the Indian reader will be more familiar with the concepts dealt with in these terms through his or her mother tongue than some approximate English equivalent. It, however, does not shirk from the responsibility of translation, adding English equivalents in footnotes accompanying the text and a 'Glossary and Index' at its end. Secondly, most of the available translations attempt a free adaptation from the aphoristic Sanskrit original, creating their own syntax, thereby violating one of the basic requirements of a good translation — that of sticking as closely as possible to the original textual structure. This work, on the other hand, sticks rigorously to the original, translating only what is stated in the concerned *sūtra*-s. When, for the sake of syntactic coherence, any extra word has been used in the translation, it has been put in brackets, to distinguish it from the words that actually occur in the original. Finally, most of the existing translations, be they of orientalist or revivalist dispositions, have one agenda — that of making an otherwise strictly technical manualistic philosophical treatise appear mystical, quasi-religious and obscure. This is achieved primarily through elaborate commentaries, which deviate immensely from the precision of the original text. Accordingly, this translation does away with any commentary providing for the student reader the original text and nothing more, from which he or she can draw independent conclusions. However, to set a perspective, the volume does include two essays — a prefatory one by Prof. Kapoor, where Yoga philosophy is set in relation to the other five orthodox systems of classical Indian philosophy, and an appendical one by me, which looks into how this philosophy deals with the important issues of cognition and signification — but one may notice how the emphasis in both is to demystify Yoga and make it the subject of serious academic studies.

Finally, after having stated the purpose of this book, I would like to thank those without whose inspiration, co-operation and support this volume would have never been possible, irrespective of its noble aims. I thank Prof. Kapoor for inspiring me and many of my likes to develop a keen interest in classical Indian philosophy, and also for having contributed a most illuminating essay as the curtain-raiser to this book. I thank D.K. Printworld for choosing to publish this manuscript, as without their support it would have been relegated to the ever-increasing heap of stillborn dreams. I thank all my friends, without whose co-operation this translation would not have taken shape, it being primarily a product of group activity. Finally, I thank my dearest Simi for having kindled and kept alive the fire in me, in whose flames only I could re-forge a project five years too old.

New Delhi, 2000 **Saugata Bhaduri**

Contents

The Śāstra Group at Jawaharlal Nehru University

— An Introduction —

AT the Centre of Linguistics and English, Jawaharlal Nehru university, beginning in 1978, a conscious decision was taken to introduce courses in the Indian intellectual traditions in grammar, literary theory and philosophy so that the young post-graduates and research students who come to J.N.U., who are among the brightest minds in the country, are in a position to interact meaningfully with the western thought and on level ground. This intellectual tradition, we know, had three main contending schools of thought — the Brahmin (also called the Grammarians), the Buddhist and the Jaina. The Brahmin School, the Grammarians, were divided into *āstika* (orthodox) and *nāstika* (heterodox) schools. These three traditions are enshrined mainly in Sanskrit and also in Pāli (Buddhist) and Prākṛta (Jaina). All the streams composed their major texts in Sanskrit which for more than 3000 years has continued to be the language of learning and scholarship in India. These three traditions, contrary to the popular perception, continue to be living traditions though through exigencies of history they have become relatively restricted to some traditional centres and institutes of learning. But the tradition is alive — this tradition of knowledge may be compared to a river, the *Gaṅgā pravāha*, which sometimes and/or at some places becomes narrow and elsewhere and at another time is a broad free flowing stream.

The task is to make this learning a part of the main-stream education, to establish a bridge between the wealth of scholarship in this tradition and the new centres of learning, the Indian universities. How is this to be achieved?

It can be achieved by making the seminal texts of the Indian intellectual traditions widely and inexpensively available. For this, we have —

1. to prepare editions of seminal intellectual texts *in different scripts*,
2. to translate/re-translate the seminal texts into English and into major Indian languages (and into major European languages), and prepare careful modern translations in contemporary idiom,
3. to expound the important theoretical frameworks in a modern idiom to bring out their contemporary relevance.

In this perspective, and with this end in view, the Centre of Linguistics and English, Jawaharlal Nehru University, New Delhi, had introduced courses first in the Indian intellectual traditions in grammar, literary theory and philosophy and then courses in the seminal texts — the grammar of Pāṇini, *Aṣṭādhyāyī*, Bharata's *Nāṭyaśāstra*, Bhartṛhari's *Vākyapadīya* and Patañjali's *Yogasūtra*. *Aṣṭādhyāyī* is studied as a primary modeling device of knowledge; *Nāṭyaśāstra* is studied as a text of communication; *Vākyapadīya* is unrivaled as a text of philosophy of language; and, *Yogasūtra* is a text of cognition and cognitive processes. This, over the years, then led in due time to considerable expositional and comparative research by a growing body of brilliant young boys and girls who, with their minds engaged by the powerful texts, became deeply involved in and committed to the Indian traditions of thought and became convinced that the theoretical frameworks of this tradition can be meaningfully related to both the contemporary Indian realities and the modern western thought.

These young scholars decided to form a group devoted to the task of opening out the Indian thought by (i) translating the seminal texts, (ii) writing expository commentaries on those texts, and (iii) applying the Indian theoretical frameworks to modern Indian and Western texts to show the power, validity and in-built development potential of these frameworks. This group, called **The Śāstra Group**, coordinated by me, has these founding members:

1. Ananya Vajpeyi
2. Anuradha Ghosh
3. Atanu Bhattacharya
4. Debashish Chakravarti
5. Gaurhari Behera
6. Mayurika Chakravarti
7. Nabanita Banerjee
8. Nalini M. Ratnam
9. Nitoo Das
10. Rajnish Kumar Mishra
11. Sadhana Parashar
12. Saugata Bhaduri
13. Shankaranarayanan
14. Shruti Pant
15. Sunita Murmu
16. Sushant Kumar Mishra
17. Swati Mustafi
18. Simi Malhotra

Objectives of Śāstra Group

1. to prepare inexpensive script variants of principal intellectual texts in the major Indian scripts,
2. to prepare modern translations of these texts in major Indian languages and produce both inexpensive student editions of each and multilingual CD texts,
3. to apply the Indian theoretical frameworks contemporary Indian texts and texts of other cultures,
4. to explore the possibility of producing reference bibliography of Sanskrit studies around the globe,
5. to prepare multi-lingual glossaries of intellectual terms in grammar, literary theory and philosophy, and
6. to start a *Journal of Indic Studies*.

The following texts have been identified in the first instance:

I. Grammar and Phonetics

1. Aṣṭādhyāyī
2. Vājasaneyi Prātiśākhya
3. Pāṇinīya Śikṣā
4. 1st Āhnika of Mahābhāṣya

II. Literary Theory

5. Bharata's Nāṭyaśāstra 6. Bhāmaha's Kāvyālaṁkāra
7. Daṇḍin's Kāvyādarśa 8. Mahimabhaṭṭa's Vyaktiviveka
9. Rājaśekhara's Kāvyamīmāṁsā
10. Anandavardhana's Dhvanyāloka
11. Abhinavagupta's Abhinavabhāratī
12. Viśvanātha's Sāhityadarpaṇa
13. Pt. Jagannātha's Rasagaṅgādhara

III. Philosophy

14. Mīmāṁsāsūtra 15. Nyāyasūtra
16. Sāṁkhyasūtra 17. Vaiśeṣikasūtra
18. Yogasūtra 19. Vedāntasūtra
20. Madhvācārya's Sarvadarśanasaṁgraha
21. Tattvārthasūtra 22. Dharmakīrti's Pramāṇavārttika
23. Jagadīśa's Śabdaśakti-prakāśikā

Some texts have already been translated — those at serial nos. 5, 6, 9, 14, 15, 16, 17, 18, 19. Other are awaiting finalisation for publication. Besides, several research studies have been completed that expound the Indian theoretical frameworks and apply them to modern texts in a significant reversal of the existing data-theory relationship.

Rajnish Kumar Mishra's exposition of *Buddhist Theory of Meaning* was the first **Śāstra Group** research belonging to the 3rd part of the Objectives to be published in the ŚĀSTRA GROUP SERIES. Based on wide-ranging primary sources, including the Buddhist philosophical-epistemological texts in Sanskrit, the book sheds altogether new light on the Buddhist theory of meaning and, simultaneously argues against the fallacies that have cropped up around its latter-day interpretations. This book has great contemporary relevance for the post-structuralist debates.

Sadhna Parashar's translation of Rājaśekhara's *Kāvyamīmāṁsā* was published as the second Śāstra Group

Publication. *Kāvyamīmāṁsā* is a seminal ninth century text of literary theory; and it is different from the preceding texts in that for the first time, various issues and dimensions of literary creativity and composition are taken up for close analysis. The discussion is of great contemporary interest and is pertinent to issues of contemporary literary theory as well. This is the only complete translation of this important text and has for years been used by succeeding batches of students in the Centre of Linguistics and English. This book will, hopefully, lead to a renewal of Rājaśekhara studies and a revival of interest in related issues.

And now, the third book, Patañjali's *Yoga-sūtras*, is being published in the Śāstra Group Series. *Yoga-sūtras* is basically, not about physical disciplining of the body, as has been popularly construed. It is a text of cognitive psychology, dealing with questions of knowledge — its nature, formation and validation. It is a short text but difficult to translate. Saugata Bhaduri has done a brilliant translation, noteworthy for its exactness and thoroughness.

I am very happy that this third volume has now been published in the Śāstra Group Series and it is a matter of great pride and satisfaction for me.

I am thankful to Jawaharlal Nehru University for providing a token amount for finalizing the manuscript.

Prof. Kapil Kapoor
Professor of English and Rector
Jawaharlal Nehru University
New Delhi - 110 067

Introduction

Yoga philosophy is one of the six orthodox schools of Indian philosophy and it is closely associated with Sāṁkhya. The first thing one should look into, to understand what the philosophy is all about, is the etymological meaning of the word *yoga*. The word is normally used to mean 'conjunction' but Vācaspatimiśra commenting on I.1. of *Yoga-sūtra* in his *Tattvavaiśāradī* says that *yoga*, in the sense it is used in this philosophy, comes from √*yuj-a* (*Dhātupāṭha*, IV.68) meaning 'concentration' (as seen in words like *yukti*), and not from √*yuj-i* (*Dhātupāṭha*, VII.7) meaning 'conjunction'. In connection with the Western languages, it can be shown how *yoga* in this sense has more to do with the English 'yoke', whereby one gains power and control over something, and less with the Greek *zygon* or the Latin *jugum* and their English derivatives like 'conjugation'. *Yoga* philosophy is thus about gaining control over oneself, and his or her surroundings, in order to gain 'liberation'.

Yoga can be of various types — *rāja-yoga*, *karma-yoga*, *jñāna-yoga*, *dhyāna-yoga*, and even *haṭha-yoga* which deals with physical exercises. The tradition of philosophical texts of the system deals, however, with *dhyāna-yoga*, or the achievement of *yoga* through *dhyāna*,[1] alone. Our discussion will accordingly be restricted to this only.

As we have already said, Yoga is closely related to Sāṁkhya. It accepts the Sāṁkhya epistemology whereby the *citta*, because of cognition (mostly through perception), develops *vṛtti*-s whose

---

1. All the Saṁskṛta technical terms used in the 'Introduction' may be checked in the 'Index' for their meanings and their occurrences in the primary text.

nirodha is imperative for attaining *viveka-jñāna* (discriminating knowledge), which is essential to liberation. Yoga, as a system, provides the means to this attainment. It says that among the five types of *citta* shown by Sāṁkhya, it is not possible to perform *yoga* in the first three of *kṣipta* (excited), *mūḍha* (unintelligent) and *vikṣipta* (fragmented) kinds, but the fourth type of *ekāgra-citta* (singly intent) sets *yoga* in motion and the fifth — *niruddha-citta* — is that state which the means are to achieve.

Yoga accepts the Sāṁkhya ontology of 25 principles also, but adds one more category of *īśvara* to them, forming a major difference with the latter. The Yoga system gives two prime reasons for its becoming *seśvara* or theistic. First, anything which has degrees must have a limit too, and thus knowledge, which proceeds in degrees, has to have an ultimate omniscience to it — which is *īśvara*. Secondly, neither *prakṛti* nor *puruṣa* having the properties of association or dissociation, the evolution of this world from their association, and its dissolution from their dissociation, must have an agency behind them, namely *īśvara*.

Apart from the concept of *īśvara*, the Yoga system, adding nothing new to Sāṁkhya philosophy, it is less of a *śāstra* and more of, as *Yoga-sūtra* itself acknowledges in I.1, an *anuśāsana* or discipline. The system teaches how through the observance of the eight *aṅga*-s of *yama*, *niyama*, *āsana*, *prāṇāyāma*, *pratyāhāra*, *dhāraṇā*, *dhyāna* and *samādhi*, one can perform *yoga*. This may be either *samprajñāta* (conscious of objects) or *asamprajñāta*. The former being achievable through *vitarka*, *vicāra, ānanda* and *asmitā* also, it is the latter which is more conducive to the liberative end. The final stage of *samādhi* is primarily *sabīja* (with seeds for producing *saṁskāra*-s) leaving behind one final *saṁskāra*. A *nirodha* of this also leads to the ultimate stage of *nirbīja* or 'seedless' *samādhi*. Here, all *citta-vṛtti*-s having dwindled away, the *puruṣa* and *sattva* are no longer confused to be one and the same, and the *ātmā* gets ready for *kaivalya* or liberation.

The primary text of Yoga philosophy is Patañjali's *Yoga-sūtra* which has four books and a total of 195 *sūtra*-s, and a translation of this follows. Other important texts in the tradition are Vyāsa's commentary *Yoga-bhāṣya*, Vācaspatimiśra's sub-commentary *Tattva-vaiśāradī*, Bhojarāja's simple and popular expositions — *Vitti* and *Yoga-maṇiprabhā*, and Vijñānabhikṣu's manuals — *Yoga-vārttika* and *Yogasāra-saṁgraha*, which have often been consulted to understand the philosophy, but have not been included in the translation.

Six Indian Philosophical Systems and Patañjali's Yoga-sūtras

Indian philosophical systems

THE word used for **philosophy** is *darśana* from the Sanskrit root *dṛś* which means 'to see' — **philosophy** means 'love of argument' and suggests an effort to impose a framework on the visible world/reality in order to make sense of it. *Darśana*, on the other hand, accords no constructive role to man's mind and means 'observation of things the way they are', to see them for what they are. As such it is very much an empirical inquiry and, contrary to the popular perception, its concerns are very concrete and this-worldly.

Indian philosophical systems fall into three schools — the brāhmaṇa (also called, in the tradition, the grammarians), the Buddhists and the Jains. The different philosophical systems can also be classified as (i) *āstika* (orthodox), and (ii) *nāstika* (heterodox). The parameter of orthodoxy, however, is different — acceptance of *śruti*s (Vedas) as *pramāṇa* (valid epistemology) is the criterion. Thus the Cārvāka, the Buddhist and the Jain systems are considered heterodox on this count. Three of the six orthodox schools — Mīmāṁsā, Vedānta, Sāṁkhya, Yoga, Vaiśeṣika, Nyāya — Mīmāṁsā, Sāṁkhya and Vaiśeṣika are *nirīśvara* (godless) schools, that is they do not posit 'god' as an ontological category and yet they are *āstika* because they accept Vedas as valid epistemology.

For each philosophical system, there is an authoritative text bearing the same name as the philosophical system itself and associated with a celebrated thinker as the author — Jaimini's *Mīmāṁsa-sūtra*, Bādarāyaṇa's *Vedānta-sūtra*, Kapila's *Saṁkhya-sūtra*, Patañjali's *Yoga-sūtra*, Kaṇāda's *Vaiśeṣika-sūtra*, Gautama's *Nyāya-sūtra*. We do not know when these texts were composed but it is safe to assume that they were composed in that age of empire building from 1000 BC onwards which was a period of great vigour and intellectual ferment and saw the formation of both political empires and intellectual systems. It is in this period that Pāṇini's *Aṣṭādhyāyī* was composed and in this age Buddha propounded his philosophy of useful action and good reason. These philosophical systems are the reasoned answers to some basic questions related to this **human** life in this world, questions that has been examined in a long tradition of philosophical inquiry that had its origins in the Upaniṣads.

Every system has a *sūtra* (text consisting of aphoristic statements), a *bhāṣya* (commentary) and a *vārttika* (elucidation of the commentary). A *sūtra* text states its truths in an extremely terse form so that the small text can be held in the mind. For this reason, it needs to be elucidated. The commentaries apart from explaining the text with examples often extend and enrich the original text and are studied as extensions of the original text. Thus, for example, the *Pūrva Mīmāṁsā-sūtra* is by Jaimini, its *Bhāṣya* by Śabarasvāmin and its *Vārttika* by Kumārilabhaṭṭa.

Purpose and nature of philosophical inquiry: Overcoming suffering

It has been said, and it is widely believed, that the concerns of Indian philosophy are purely metaphysical and that their ultimate goal is to facilitate the achievement of *mokṣa* which is often translated as 'salvation'. Now the agenda of Indian systems, both theistic and atheistic, is the same — to find an answer to the problem of suffering of this, and in this, worldly life. The inquiry concerns this life and if some systems propound some metaphysical ontological categories like 'self' (*ātman*), 'the great self' (*paramātman*), etc., they argue that these are **real** instruments of alleviation of worldly suffering.

So the basic question that is addressed is the question of *duḥkha*, suffering. As is declared by the *Sāṁkhya-sūtra*,[1] the goal of human life (*puruṣārtha*) is to seek liberation (*nivṛtti*) from the three kinds of suffering — accidental, bodily, spiritual. We can do nothing about accidental suffering — an earthquake, for example. For bodily suffering, ailments of the body, the *Caraka-saṁhitā*, a text of *Āyurveda*, says we need *cikitsā*, medicinal treatment and for spiritual/mental suffering we need to study *darśana*, philosophy.

So the philosophical systems are each a different answer to this question of mental/spiritual suffering. All systems argue that **right knowledge** is the supreme means of liberation — they differ on the nature of this 'right knowledge'. But they all agree that this has to be a cognition of some ontological and epistemological truths by an individual knowing self. It is this awareness of what it is that immunes man to suffering, that makes him immune to those **causes** that make a man suffer. Suffering is inevitable — all that one can seek is the wisdom to rationalise suffering and reduce its potential to damage the self.

The different systems — Ontology and epistemology

The word *veda* is from the verb-root *vid* which means 'to see'/'to know'.[2] *Veda* therefore means 'knowledge' and it is assumed to be non-contingent knowledge, that is knowledge free of time, place, individual. Vedic literature is classified into three broad divisions — *Mantras*, *Brāhmaṇas* and *Upaniṣads*.

The knowledge embodied in these texts has been systematised and analysed by various thinkers and presented in the primary philosophical texts enumerated above. *Darśana*, philosophy, is defined as — *dṛśyate anena iti darśanam*, that is

---

1. *Sāṁkhya-sūtra*, 1.1.ff.
2. The same proto-Indo-European root *vid* underlies the English words 'visual'/'visualise'. The word 'seer' is an exact analogue of the Sanskrit word *draṣṭā* both with the meaning 'a wiseman who apprehends knowledge directly'.

'with the help of which the essential self (*tāttvika svarūpa*) of something is seen'. What is the starting point of Indian philosophy? Its meta-assumption is that all living beings tend towards *duḥkha-nivṛtti* (freedom from suffering).

So philosophy addresses the question of *duḥkha* (suffering). It concerns itself with four related issues:

(i) *heya* — the real nature of *duḥkha* (suffering).

(ii) *heyahetu* — the real cause of suffering.

(iii) *hāna* — what is the complete absence of suffering; what is that condition?

(iv) *hānopāya* — what is the means/method of achieving the complete absence of suffering.

In the examination of these questions, three ontological entities present themselves:

(i) *Cetana-tattva* — the life principle variously called *ātmā*, *puruṣa* (*jīva*). The question — who suffers? What is the nature of the one who suffers? Is suffering its natural property? The argument is that once one is face to face with this real self, one is in the state of complete absence of suffering, *hāna*.

(ii) *Jaḍa-tattva* — inert matter, *prakṛti*. That in which suffering originates, of which suffering is the necessary attribute. Not being able to distinguish between this inert matter and the life principle is the cause of suffering, *heyahetu*. Discriminating knowledge that enables a distinction between this and the life principle is the means of putting an end of suffering, *hānopāya*.

(iii) *Cetanā-tattva* — the great Self, variously called *paramātmā*, *īśvara*, *brahman*. That which is the goal of the individual self, becoming one with which the individual self becomes autonomous of the inert matter and therefore immune to suffering.

In order to explain these four substantial concepts, the

Śāstras, philosophical texts, explain the three *tattva*s, ontological entities, in precise, logical statements. Six of these philosophical systems are: Mīmāṁsā, Vedānta, Nyāya, Vaiśeṣika, Sāṁkhya, Yoga. These six are considered auxiliary to the study of Vedas. They are customarily classed into three sets of two related systems — Mīmāṁsā and Vedānta (Pūrva Mīmāṁsā and Uttara Mīmāṁsā); Vaiśeṣika and Nyāya; Sāṁkhya and Yoga.

Mīmāṁsā and Vedānta

Vedas teach three ways of living one's life: *karma-kāṇḍa* (the path of enjoined action); *upāsanā-kāṇḍa* (the path of devotion); *jñāna-kāṇḍa* (the path of knowledge).

Mīmāṁsā, known as Pūrva-Mīmāṁsā is the largest text — it has 2644 *sūtra*s and 909 topics (*adhikaraṇa*). Its number of *sūtras* is equal to those of the other five put together. In its 12 chapters it analyses *dharma*, which is announced as its subject by the very first *sūtra* — *athāto dharmajijñāsā*, 'heretofore, we investigate what is *dharma*'. According to Mīmāṁsā, *dharma* consists in the performance of enjoined actions by doing which one is able to sever the relation of self (*ātmā*) with the body, the senses and the objects of senses. Therefore, Mīmāṁsā teaches *karma-kāṇḍa*, the manifold path of action; it teaches —

(i) *nitya-karma*, acts that should be performed everyday.

(ii) *naimittika-karma*, acts to be performed when some event takes place, like the birth of a child.

(iii) *kāmya-karma*, acts performed with some worldly or other-worldly end in view.

There are two other kinds of acts:

(iv) *niṣiddha-karma*, proscribed actions, acts proscribed by the Śāstras, and

(v) *prāyaścitta-karma*, acts performed to cleans one's self of the impressions (*saṁskāra*s) left on the self by an indulgence in proscribed actions.

Maharṣi Jaimini says performance of the enjoined acts with faith would lead to 'heaven', bliss, here and now. Mīmāṁsā asserts that all knowledge is self-validated, for knowledge takes form only when necessary and sufficient conditions are present. Mīmāṁsā epistemology allows perception, inference, verbal authority (*śabda pramāṇa*), implication (*arthāpatti*). The Prābhākara School accepts analogy (*upamāna*) as the fifth epistemology. The (Kumārila) Bhāṭṭa School accepts in addition non-presence (*anupalabdhi*) as the sixth epistemology.

Mīmāṁsā accepts the externally existing world as real, accepts the material reality but does not accept a god (*paramātmā* or *īśvara*) as the creator ot this universe which, Mīmāṁsā says, has always existed and therefore this universe (*jagat*) has had no beginning (*anādi*) and no end (*ananta*). Action is an independent power and it makes the world go.

Vedānta, also known as Uttara Mīmāṁsā, is expressed in the Sūtras known varioulsy as *Brahma-sūtra*, *Śārīrika-sūtra*, *Vedānta-sūtra* attributed to Vyāsa known in the tradition as Bādarāyaṇa. Uttara Mīmāṁsā teaches the path of knowledge, the knowledge of *Brahman* as its very first *sūtra* declares — *athāto brahmanjijñāsā*, 'heretofore we investigate what is *brahman*'. The topics treated are — *īśvara* (god), *prakṛti* (matter), *jīvātmā* (individual life principle), *punarjanma* (re-birth), states after death, *karma* (action), *upāsanā* (devotion/worship), *jñāna* (knowledge), *bandha* (bondage), *mokṣa* (liberation). Vedānta says suffering is the property of the material body (*jaḍa-tattva*), ignorance in the form of imposition of the body on the self (*ātmā*) is its cause, delinking one's self completely from the material body and establishing oneself in one's self constitutes the state of total absence of suffering, and to achieve this establishment in one's self, one must gain knowledge of the Great/Universal Self/Life Principle (*paramātmava-tattva*) which is totally alien to the principle of sorrow. The grand opposition of *dvaita~advaita* (dualism~non-dualism) concerns the relationship between the Individual Self and the Universal Self — in the state of *hāna* (complete absence of suffering), the two are argued to remain separate (dualism) or become one (non-dualism).

The central concept of Vedānta is *Brahman*. Sāṁkhya had posited two ultimate ontological categories — *prakṛti* (matter) and *puruṣa* (energy). Vedānta captures with great insight the fact that energy is not separate from but is in fact immanent in matter. *Brahman* is this one principle which subsumes both energy and matter. As such it is described in *Vedānta-sūtra*s as the substratum, the cause and the pervasive principle of the entire universe. This construct establishes the oneness of all being — the multiplicity (*nānātva*) and difference exist at the level of appearance. The source of this construct is to be found in the *Ṛgveda*, *puruṣasūkta* which conceives of a *puruṣa* which permeates the entire *brahmāṇḍa* (universe) and even beyond and all the inert and living entities are seen as parts or forms of that.

The first four *sūtra*s called *catuḥsūtrī* (1.1.1-4) generally state the substance of this concept of *Brahman*; the rest of the text is an explication. It is said —

> Now we will investigate *Brahman* (1.1.1); that which is the efficient cause (*nimitta*) of the origin, maintenance and destruction of this universe is *Brahman* (1.1.2); *Brahman* is established/proved by sister (1.1.3); the purpose of *śruti*s is establishment of *Brahman* (1.1.4).

This *Brahman* is described in its two aspects — in (a) its formless, attributeless (*nirguṇa*) aspect, and (b) its manifest (*saguṇa*) aspect. In its pure, attributeless, formless (*nirguṇa*) aspect, the non-manifest (*avyakta*) *Brahman* is beyond the dichotomy of form~formless (3.2.23).

Vedānta originated in the Upaniṣads but has continuously been commented upon and developed. Later a number of thinkers wrote their commentaries upon Jaimini's *sūtra*s and extended this system of thought. The greatest of them all, of course, is Ādi Śaṅkara who in his celebrated *Śārīrika-bhāṣya* established his non-dualist (*advaita*) principle:

(i) The multiplicity of the visible world is only a reflex of the one attributeless essence (*tattva*).

(ii) Inherent in the *Brahman* is its creative power (*māyā*) by which it appears in various manifest forms as so many objects.

(iii) So *Brahman* with its creative power (*māyā*) is the efficient cause of this universe.

(iv) The individual due to ignorance (*avidyā*), confuses his real self with his material body.

(v) On gaining knowledge of the oneness of *Brahman* and *ātmā* (*brahmātmaikatva*), the self-ness in the material body is lost leading to the extinction of *kartā-bhoktā* (doer-experiencer) awareness which in its turn frees man from the effect of his actions ending in his liberation from suffering.

The eleventh-century savant, Śrī Rāmānujācārya, the next great Vedānta-exegete modified the Śaṅkara principle by arguing the reality of the visible, material world. His principle has come to be known as Viśiṣṭādvaita. The third great original Vedānta-exegete is Śrī Madhvācārya who argued that the Universal Self (*Brahman*) and the Individual Self (*jīva*) are two different entities and consistently remain so. And as with Śrī Rāmānujācārya, the Madhvācārya principle accords primacy to *saguṇa* (manifest) divinity (*īśvara*) and therefore his followers are believers in ritual worship.

Vedānta, particularly Śaṅkara's *Advaita Vedānta* has had a very wide and deep influence on Indian life.

Nyāya and Vaiśeṣika

These two systems have much in common. The Vaiśeṣika system concerns itself with ontology and Nyāya, accepting Vaiśeṣika ontology concerns itself with epistemological issues. The number of *Vaiśeṣika-sūtra*s is 370 divided into ten chapters with two *āhnika*s (sections) in each chapter. The first part of the first chapter describes the properties and divisions of substances (*dravya*), qualities (*guṇa*) and actions (*karma*). In the second part of the first chapter, the general or universal is defined. Nine substances have been described in the second and third chapters, the atom theory (*paramāṇu-vāda*) in the first part of the fourth chapter, the transient substances in the second part of the fourth chapter, acts/actions in the fifth chapter, epistemological status of the Vedas and the constructs of *dharma-adharma* in the sixth, some qualities in the seventh and the eighth chapters, absence (*abhāva*) and knowledge (*jñāna*) in the ninth chapter and *sukha-duḥkha* (joy-sorrow) difference and their causes in the tenth chapter.

The word *vaiśeṣika* means indicator of different *padārtha*s (objects). *Padārtha*s are those that one cognises by perception. Possession of the right knowledge of the six elements — substance, quality, action, universal, particular, and inseparable connection — will enable us to handle the problem of suffering. Vaiśeṣika is obviously a materialist system which posits atoms as the ultimate constituents of all objects.

Vaiśeṣika divides the object of knowledge (*prameya*), into seven *padārtha*s:

> *dravya* (substance, *guṇa* (quality), *karma* (action), *sāmānya* (association), *viśeṣa* (difference), *samavāya* (inherence) and *abhāva* (non-existence):

1. *dravya* — earth, water, fire, space, time, direction, self and mind are the nine substances.
2. *guṇa* — colour, taste, smell, touch, number, measure, separateness, conjunction, division, distant, non-distant, gravitation, fluidity, oiliness/lubricity, sound, intellect, joy, sorrow, desire, enmity/repugnance, effort, *dharma* (righteousness), *adharma* (unrighteousness), *saṁskāra* (endowed power such as speed in air, etc., state of mind, restorative power as for example a branch of a tree which is held down goes back to its original position when release).

3. *karma* — five kinds of movement: upwards, downwards, constriction, expansion and change of place/going.
4. *sāmānya* — universal of a class of objects such as **treeness** of trees.
5. *viśeṣa* — specificity or particular.
6. *samavāya* — intimate union, and
7. *abhāva* — non-presence, absence.

Nyāya, it may be noted, also accepts these ontological categories. That is why these two systems go together — in these philosophical systems, truth consists in the nature of these *padārthas*; therefore, to get to know the truth, we must go to the root of these *padārthas*. To achieve this, we must make use of all valid *pramāṇas*, means of knowledge. *Padārthas* are divided into two — 'existent' and 'non-existent': the first six of the *padārthas* listed above belong to the 'existent' category while the seventh, *abhāva*, constitutes the 'non-existent' category. Of these seven, *dravya, guṇa* and *karma* belong to the category of *sat* or 'being'; that is, we can demonstrate their existence (qualities like 'happiness' and 'redness' can be shown to be existing in substances). Existence of the other four *padārthas* cannot be demonstrated.

Nyāya also says like Vaiśeṣika that truth will be known if we have knowledge of the *padārthas* and develop detachment that will lead to release, a state in which we know neither joy nor sorrow. Nyāya is also called Tarka-Śāstra — its main purpose being to establish by reasoning that the *kartā* or creator of all this world is Parameśvara. It is in this positing of *īśvara* that Nyāya differs from Vaiśeṣika. The Nyāya inquiry into truth is through the four *pramāṇas* or instruments of knowledge — *pratyakṣa* (perception), *anumāna* (inference), *upamāna* (analogy) and *śabda* (verbal testimony). But, predominantly, both Nyāya and Vaiśeṣika **conduct** inquiries through inference. Gautama Akṣapāda's *Nyāya-sūtra* has five chapters, with two sections in each chapter, in which the definition and characteristics of the following sixteen subjects are discussed:

> Objects of knowledge, means of knowledge, doubt, purpose, analogy, conclusion, part of a logical argument, argument, judgement, disputation (*vāda*), debate (*jalpa*), fallacious argument (*vitaṇḍa*), fallacious middle term (*hetvābhāsa*), deception, class, a fault in syllogism.

With proper knowledge of these sixteen objects, the self transcends hunger-thirst, greed-infatuation (*lobha-moha*), cold-heat and becomes liberated (*mukta*) and in that state joy-sorrow become non-existent. And this knowledge is attained by four means of knowledge — perception, inference, analogy and verbal testimony.

The basic principle of both Nyāya and Vaiśeṣika is *kārya-kāraṇa-vāda* (cause-effect theory) also called *paramāṇu-vāda* (atomist theory) which asserts that everything that exists has a prior cause. The ultimate cause or constituents of all gross material objects are subtle sub-atomic particles (*paramāṇu*). The conjunction of these particles in a hierarchic structure is accepted by these systems as the material cause of this visible universe. Of course, senses and *īśvara* are accepted as the two instrumental or efficient causes.

> Nyāya or Tarka (logic) gives rationalism its due place, but this does not lead to materialism, atheism or the Lokāyata system. Through intellectual inquiry, Nyāya comes to the conclusion that, if the world is so orderly with so many creatures in it, all of them interlinked, there must be an *īśvara* to have created it. Nyāya recognises that there are areas that cannot be comprehended by human reason and that the truths that cannot be established rationally must be accepted according to how Vedas see them. . . . Instead of idling away one's time without making any intellectual effort to discover the truth, would it not be better to keep thinking about things it be to arrive at the conclusion that there is no God? A person who does so is superior to the idler who has no intellectual concern whatsoever.

Perhaps the atheist, were he to continue his inquiry, would develop sufficient intellectual clarity to give up his atheism. But the idler has no means of advancing inwardly.

This is one reason why even 'Cārvākam' was accepted as a system. . . . Cārvākam believes that there is no need to worry about god or any spirit or to observe vows and fasts or to control one's senses. Live as you please according to your whims and according to the dictates of your senses.[3]

Sāṁkhya and Yoga

These two, says the *Bhagavad Gītā*, are the two most ancient systems and standing respectively for the paths of knowledge and of action. The first *sūtra* of Sāṁkhya says that as the proper knowledge of *tattvas* (the ontological entities) is the means of liberation from suffering, we will investigate what these *tattvas* are. As against the principle of intelligence that desires freedom from suffering, there is/must be the principle of matter, *prakṛti*, and the second and the third *sūtras* described the eight-fold *prakṛti* and the sixteen *vikāras*. Inert matter has two aspects — *prakṛti* (unmodified) and *vikṛti* (modified). That from which some other element is born is *prakṛti* and that finally formed element from which no other element can be born is *vikṛti*. After noting the 24 unmodified and the modified ontological elements, the fourth *sūtra* enunciates *puruṣa* as the twenty-fifth element, the 'intelligence'/'life' principle. The fifth *sūtra* (*traiguṇyam*) enunciates the all important doctrine of three-fold *prakṛti*, that three innate propensities (determining properties) belong to all the 24 elements.

The three *guṇas* are *sattva*, *rajas*, *tamas* and in each ontological substance, modified and unmodified, one of these

3. Pujyasri Chandrasekhara Sarasvati Svami, *Hindu Dharma. The Universal Way of Life*, Bombay: Bharartiya Vidya Bhavan, pp. 419-20.

three properties predominates and the predominating property determines the nature and state of that substance. These *guṇa*s are dynamic principles and continually bring about change and produce result in and from the substances — they bring about the creation (*sṛṣṭi*) and destruction (*pralaya*). These three 'qualities' are accepted by all systems. *Sattva* denotes a state of perfection, of goodness, clarity, and serenity; *rajas* is all action, movement and passion; *tamas* is inertia, sloth and darkness. Sāṁkhya believes that in all beings a balance obtains among these three 'forces' and when an imbalance develops, undesirable consequences follow. This balance obtains in individuals, in 'systems', social, political, etc., and in the cosmos. This balance is the *ṛta* of the *Ṛgveda*. When this is disturbed, changes follow, desirable and undesirable, new elements may be formed, new conditions and factors come into play and there is great, restless flux till a new balance is achieved, that is the three inherent forces acquire a new equipoise. But Sāṁkhya does not tell us how this is to be achieved — through worship of *īśvara*, inquiry into one's self or through performance of enjoined actions. It does not go beyond telling us to be aware of the difference between the 'alert intelligence' (*puruṣa*) and 'inert matter' (*prakṛti*).

Yoga

It is Patañjali's Yoga system that informs us of the practical means of dissociating the Self, the alert intelligence or life principle from the inert matter, of the *sādhanā* to be followed to become aware of the difference. The concept of *īśvara*, absent in Sāṁkhya, is central in Yoga and devotion is an important construct in the method of bringing the mind under control.

There is much in common between Sāṁkhya and Yoga which accepts the 25 ontological elements. According to Sāṁkhya, a discriminating intellect is the instrument of liberation and this discriminating intellect is acquired only through the practice of *yoga*. What is *yoga*? *Yoga* is control of the tendency of the experiencing self to attach itself to the external objects so that the experiencing self (*citta*) becomes stabilised in its basic/native condition.

Yoga-sūtra has 159 *sūtras* in four chapters. The first chapter, *Samādhipāda*, describes the nature of *yoga* and this is explained in the three *sūtras* 2-4, the rest of the chapter being an explication of these three statements. "*Yoga* is control of the activity of the experiencing self" (1.1.2); "In that state of control the experiencer is established in his native self" (1.1.3); "Else, the experiencer becomes one with the activity of the self" (1.1.4). Stability of the mind or the self, its one-pointedness or focusing on **one** something (*ekāgratā*) is the great secret. *Ekāgratā* is keeping the mind engrossed in one thought to the exclusion of every other thought. The mind can focus on —

1. gross object,
2. subtle object/thought,
3. one's conscious self,
4. the inner self.

Unless the mind is so stabilised, the self will remain disturbed (*vikṣipta*) like the image of moon in turbulent water.

In the second chapter, *Sādhanapāda*, the method of regaining peace is laid down for those with *vikṣipta* (disturbed) self. Five causes of all suffering are enumerated —

1. ignorance (*avidyā*),
2. non-distinction between the material body and the self (*asmitā*),
3. desire for joys of the material body (*rāga*),
4. sorrows springing from non-fulfilment of material joys (*dveṣa*),
5. desire to protect the body for suffering (*abhiniveśa*).

Possible suffering should be renounced. The conjunction of the seer (*dṛṣṭa*) and what is there to see (*dṛśya*) is the cause of suffering. (2.16, 17) What is there to see? All this visible world (the 24 elements of Sāṁkhya) which is characterised by three-fold properties. The seer (*dṛṣṭa*) though intrinsically pure in its native self is permeated by the activities (*vṛttis*) of the experiencing self. The indiscriminate coming together of the seer and the seen is due to lack of true knowledge or understanding. When one overcomes ignorance, one overcomes indiscriminate conjunction and that produces the absence of suffering. One overcomes ignorance by the highest form of discriminating intellect (*viveka-khyāti*). What is this high state of the Intellect (*prajñā*)? In this state —

1. All that was there to know has been known.
2. Whatever was to be distanced has been distanced.
3. Whatever was to be witnessed has been witnessed.
4. Whatever had to be done has been done; nothing more remains to be done.
5. The experiencing self has earned its right to liberation and no more right is there to be earned.
6. The properties of the experiencing self after fulfilling indulgence and liberation are beginning to dissolve back into their causes.
7. Free from the *guṇas*, the experiencing self is preparing to assimilate itself with the great Self.

In *sūtras* 29 to 55 of the second chapter, the five steps that constitute the outer phase of *yoga* are laid out. *Yama* is "abstaining from violence, stealing, covetousness and telling truth and continence". (2.29) *Niyama* is "purity, austerity, contentment, repetition of sacred words, devotion to God". (2.32) *Āsana* implies steadiness and comfort. (2.46) Control of breath, of exhalation and inhalation is *prāṇāyāma*. (2.49) *Pratyāhāra* is "the restoration of sense to the original purity of mind by renouncing its objects". (2.54)

The third chapter, *Vibhūtipāda*, describes the other three steps, *dhāraṇā*, *dhyāna* and *samādhi*, together called *saṁyama*.

"Attention fixed upon an object is *dhāraṇā*." (3.1) "Union of mind and object is *dhyāna*." (3.2) *Samādhi* is that condition of illumination where union as union disappears, only the experience of the object on which the attention is fixed being present." (3.3) In *dhāraṇā*, the attention upon an object is disturbed; in *dhyāna*, the attention is not disturbed, but the consciousness of the thinker, the thinking and the object of thought are present; in *samādhi*, separate consciousness of the thinker, the thinking, the separate object disappear only the object, transformed by and transparent to thought, remains. By practising these, one acquires many powers (*siddhis*), but a true practitioner does not use them for these hinder his progress towards final illumination. "These powers of knowledge are obstacles to illumination [enlightenment]; but illumination apart, they bring success." (3.37) "Finally, by renouncing even these powers, the seed of bondage being destroyed, the *yogī* attains liberation." (3.50)

The final chapter, *kaivalyapāda*, deals with the state of enlightenment/liberation. The self is freed of the agenthood, the role of the experiencer, of the participant becoming a pure observer. "He who sees clearly, refuses to identify the mind with the self." (4.25) The individual then is also freed of self-consciousness — who am I/what am I/how am I? Freed of this nothing remains to be achieved and — in the last of the nine states of consciousness described in the *Yoga-sūtras* — the *guṇas* (the three qualities of being) dissolve in their own substratum/cause and this is liberation, the full revelation of the power of the self, its being only itself (*kaivalya*). (4.34) "Mind without impurity and impediment, attains infinite knowledge; what is worth knowing in this world becomes negligible." (4.31)

The answers to the question — How to get rid of suffering, here and now

Two questions are central to all philosophical inquiry — the nature and status of the universe, *jagat*, its materiality and its ultimate, 'total' reality, and secondly the relationship between man, his happiness, and this universe. As we noted at length in 1994,[4] each philosophical system asserts that a valid knowledge of this total reality is the most efficacious means of achieving *mokṣa*, liberation which in final terms amounts to freedom from suffering. Each system gives its own definition of this required knowledge. Mīmāṁsā asserts that it consists in the proper performance of enjoined acts of sacrifice and duty (*karma*). But right performance is possible only after a right knowledge of objects involved in the acts. Mīmāṁsā believes in the reality of the external world (*bāhya sattā*) — reality of the physical world is a fact of perception (*pratyakṣa*) and the objects of this world are either primordial or constructs of these primordial objects. In Vedānta (Uttara Mīmāṁsā), this knowledge consists in the awareness that all the visible, diverse, multiple forms, objects both with and without life, are reflexes of the same **one** undifferentiated non-discrete Being (*sattā*) that permeates the entire universe. Sāṁkhya system describes the effort that leads to freedom from three kinds of *duḥkha* (sorrow), physical, spiritual and accidental. The effort must be directed at achieving a discriminating intellect (*viveka-jñāna*) which tells us that this entire visible creation is a product of *prakṛti* (matter) and *puruṣa* (spirit or life principle) interaction. *Prakṛti*, a modulation of 25 primordial elements, is characterised by three attributes (*guṇa*) which are in the original state but are modulated in interaction with the life-principle (*puruṣa*) so that one or the other attribute dominates and becomes the cause of suffering or happiness, as the case may be. A proper **knowledge** of *puruṣa*, the essential self, enables one to see all suffering as unrelated to this essential self. But the discriminating intellect is not sufficient to free us of suffering — we need to meditate on the primordial elements, the objects of our discriminating intellect and strive to detach/ dissociate our self from them. Yoga attributes our sorrows to

4. K. Kapoor, "Concept of *padārtha* in Language and Philosophy" in *Sir William Jones Volume Commemorating the Bicentennary of His Death* (1794-1994). Bulletin of the Deccan College Post-Graduate & Research Institute, Pune, Vols. 54-5 (1994-5), pp. 197-221.

the distractions of our *citta* and advocates, as the means of joy (*ānanda*), a disciplining of the *citta*'s potential to attach itself to objects of cognition. This disciplining depends on an understanding of the true nature of objects, on the ability to keep separate the *nāma* (designating world), *rūpa* (the form) and *jñāna* (knowledge/experience of the object). Progressively more evolved cognising consciousness, achieved through different forms of yogic meditation, enables one to achieve the discriminating intellect (*viveka-jñāna*) that frees us of the bondage of the word that filters indiscriminately into our self. Nyāya also seeks to liberate the self (*ātmā*) from the body, senses and the worldly object that constitute the objects of senses. The objects are either grasped by senses, in which case they are 'physically perceptible' or they are cognised by our mind, in which case they are 'mentally perceptible' but yet products of perception. This creation (*sṛṣṭi*) is a permutation of atoms (*paramāṇu*) and each object represents a particular permutation. Only a proper knowledge of the true nature of objects (*tattva-artha*) enables one to decide what is to be acquired or grasped and what is to be rejected and renounced. With the rise of such proper knowledge of the world, and of the self, one's self is no longer subordinate to one's consciousness and, therefore, does not experience either joy or sorrow, i.e., transcends the dichotomies and becomes one no longer subject to conflicts (*dvandvātīta*). The Vaiśeṣika system also seeks to show the path to cessation of sorrow through *tattva-jñāna*, a knowledge of the essential reality of the world. It divides all the worldly objects of knowledge into seven classes (and their sub-classes) and analyses the structure of these objects — their nature, properties and stages. The Jaina system says that *samyak-darśana*, proper and valid knowledge of the self, is the means of *mokṣa* which in the Jaina thought is the achievement of the natural pure self through a final cessation of *karma*, i.e., mental, verbal and bodily acts (see, *Tattvārtha-sūtra* 10.2). The Buddhists attribute all sorrows to 'ignorance' (*avidyā*) — the sorrows are 'real but it is possible to be unaffected by them by attaining or practising *nirvāṇa-*

mārga, which includes proper or valid knowledge as the first stage of its eight-fold path . . . .

> Therefore in all the major Indian systems of thought . . . peace and happiness is attained only when we comprehend the true nature and totality of the objects that constitute the world around us and the substance of our cognitions.[5]

This translation of Yoga-sūtra

As part of the long-term project of making available in modern translations the important texts of the Indian intellectual traditions in English and other Indian languages to students and scholars of languages, literatures and cultures, this English translation of Patañjali's *Yoga-sūtra*s is being presented as the first venture. This is an important text because it is one text that deals with the theory of knowledge — and not in the abstract but in relation to human happiness. Knowledge has always been prestiged in the Indian tradition and has been accepted as the supreme means of salvation. This text is the only one that sets out a practical method, a set of practices to develop the necessary mental sufficiency to be able to 'know' something.

The Śāstra Group at JNU has a definite policy on these 'translations'. The goal is to communicate the intent and purport of the propositions as accurately and as clearly as possible so:

1. The technical terms have been retained in the main body of the text and these have been annotated comprehensively. This is the only way as one cannot expect equivalents to exist in a language of another intellectual tradition and, in any case such approximate one-word equivalents are bound to deviate the meaning.
2. The Sanskrit śāstric texts are composed in a most economical style and therefore eschew all the features

5. *Ibid.*, pp. 199-200.

of what is called these days 'textual binding', all the explicit and implicit connections that hold between adjacent and even separated statements. These features as the traditional scholars show in their commentaries are reconstructable from the context, from an understanding of the whole text and from a knowledge of the wider context of the subject of discussion. These 'understood' interconnections are a major obstacle for a lay student/reader of today. We have made them explicit and these have been formally shown as such through devices of punctuation. This makes reading easier.

3. Care has been taken to keep the language brief, precise and simple. As far as possible, the order of statement, including the order of *pada*s (morphological constructions/words) has been paralleled to the extent that is permissible in the different language, English.

Our next step would be to bring out this text in two different ways —

(i) prepare script variants — that is, publish the original text in different Indian scripts, and

(ii) prepare 'translations' in major Indian languages.

These are our ambitious and auspicious hopes; they appear too ambitious but we are confident that this group of devoted, bright young boys and girls will fulfil this historical task. Saugata Bhaduri, the translator of this *Yoga-sūtra* text, represents in this excellent, painstaking, exact, carefully considered translation the best of this young group of intellectuals perfectly at home in both the Western and the Indian traditions. I record here my deep appreciation of the quality of his mind and of his work.

The Yoga-sūtra-s

BOOK ONE: *SAMĀDHIPĀDA*
(On Concentration)

GOAL OF CONCENTRATION (I.1-4)

1. अथ योगानुशासनम्।

   atha yogānuśāsanam ।

   Now, the discipline of *yoga* (is to be explained).

2. योगश्चित्तवृत्तिनिरोधः।

   yogaḥ-citta-vṛtti-nirodhaḥ ।[1]

   Yoga is the *nirodha* of *vṛtti*-s of the *citta*.[2]

3. तदा द्रष्टुः स्वरूपेऽवस्थानम्।

   tadā draṣṭuḥ svarūpe'vasthānam ।

   Then the seer gets situated in his *svarūpa*.[3]

4. वृत्तिसारूप्यम् इतरत्र।

   vṛtti-sārūpyam itaratra ।

   At other times (the self takes) the same form as the *vṛtti*-s.

---

1. In many cases like this, in the Roman transcript, compound words have been broken into their components, for better comprehension.
2. *nirodha* = restriction, *vṛtti* = fluctuation, *citta* = one of the three elements in one's *antaḥkaraṇa* or the cognising apparatus where imprints of perception are stored.
3. *svarūpa* = one's own essential form.

TYPES OF VṚTTI-S (I.5-11)

5. वृत्तयः पञ्चतय्यः क्लिष्टाक्लिष्टः।

vṛttayaḥ pañcatayyaḥ kliṣṭa-akliṣṭaḥ ।

Vṛtti-s are of five kinds (and are) *kliṣṭa* or *akliṣṭa.*[4]

6. प्रमाणविपर्ययविकल्पनिद्रास्मृतयः।

pramāṇa-viparyaya-vikalpa-nidrā-smṛtayaḥ ।

(They are) *pramāṇa*, *viparyaya*, *vikalpa*, sleep and *smṛti.*[5]

7. प्रत्यक्षानुमानागमहः प्रमाणानि।

pratyakṣa-anumāna-āgamaḥ pramāṇāni ।

Pratyakṣa, *anumāna* and *āgama*[6] are the *pramāṇa*-s.

8. विपर्ययो मिथ्याज्ञानमतद्रूपप्रतिष्ठम्।

viparyayo mithyā-jñānam-atadrūpa-pratiṣṭham ।

Viparyaya is a false knowledge,[7] where what (an object) is not like gets established.

9. शब्दज्ञानानुपाती वस्तुशूण्यो विकल्पः।

śabdajñāna-anupātī vastuśūṇyo vikalpaḥ ।

Vikalpa arises from linguistic consructions without any real object.[7]

10. अभावप्रत्ययालम्बन वृत्तिर्निद्रा।

abhāva-pratyaya-ālambana vṛttiḥ-nidrā ।

Sleep is the *vṛtti* based on the experience of nothingness.

---

4. *kliṣṭa* = hindered or causing hindrance, *akliṣṭa* its antonym. See II.3 for definition.
5. *pramāṇa* = valid epistemology, *viparyaya* = misconception, *vikalpa* = linguistic knowledge, *smṛti* = memory.
6. *pratyakṣa* = perception, *anumāna* = inference, *āgama* = testimonial knowledge.
7. *vikalpa* refers to cases where a word does not pertain to any real object but refers to linguistic constincts alone.

11. अनुभूतविषयासम्प्रमोषः स्मृतिः।

anubhūta-viṣaya-asampramoṣaḥ smṛtiḥ ।

Smṛti is an experienced object's not getting completely lost.

MEANS FOR THE NIRODHA OF VṚTTI-S (I.12-16)

12. अभ्यासवैराग्याभ्यां तन्निरोधः।

abhyāsa-vairāgyābhyāṁ tad-nirodhaḥ ।

Their *nirodha* (is possible) through *abhyāsa* and *vairāgya*.[8]

13. तत्र स्थितौ यत्नोऽभ्यासः।

tatra sthitau yatnaḥ-abhyāsaḥ ।

Abhyāsa is exertion (for an end) situated in this (state of *nirodha*).

14. स तु दीर्घकालनैरन्तर्यसत्कारसेवितो दृढ़भूमिः।

sa tu dīrghakāla-nairantarya-satkāra-sevito dṛḍha-bhūmiḥ ।

But this (*abhyāsa*) gains a firm rooting (only) when it is cultivated for a long period, uninterruptedly, and with attention.

15. दृष्टानुश्रविकविषयवितृष्णस्य वशीकारसंज्ञा वैराग्यम्।

dṛṣṭa-anuśravika-viṣaya-vitṛṣṇasya vaśīkāra-saṁjñā vairāgyam ।

Vairāgya is the consciousness of *vaśīkāra*[9] over (one's) thirst for visibly or audibly perceived objects.

16. तत्परंपुरुषख्यातेर्गुणवैतृष्ण्यम्।

tatparaṁ-puruṣa-khyāteḥ-guṇa-vaitṛṣṇyam ।

---

8. *abhyāsa* = practice, *vairāgya* = passionlessness/renunciation.
9. *vaśīkāra* = the power to control, to be a master of.

This is highest when *khyāti* of the *puruṣa* results in a thirstlessness for the *guṇa*-s[10] (also).

TYPES OF YOGA (I.17-20)

17. वितर्कविचारानन्दास्मितानुगमात्सम्प्रज्ञातः।

vitarka-vicāra-ānanda-asmitā-anugamāt-samprajñātaḥ ।

Samprajñāta (*yoga*) is arrived at through *vitarka*, *vicāra*, *ānanda* or *asmitā*.[11]

18. विरामप्रत्ययाभ्यासपूर्वः संस्कारशेषोऽन्यः

virāma-pratyaya-abhyāsa-purvaḥ saṁskāra-śeṣaḥ-anyaḥ ।

The other type (*asamprajñāta*[12] *yoga*) is the one which is preceded by *abhyāsa* and causes a cessation (of *vṛtti*-s), giving rise to *saṁskāra*-s[13] at the end.

19. भवप्रत्ययो विदेहप्रकृतिलयानाम्।

bhavapratyayo videha-prakṛtilayānām ।

(This *asamprajñāta yoga*) gives rise to the experience of being discarnate and dissolved in *prakṛti*.[14]

20. श्रद्धावीर्यस्मृतिसमाधिप्रज्ञापूर्वक इतरेषाम्।

śraddhā-vīrya-smṛti-samādhi-prajñā-pūrvaka itareṣām ।

---

10. *khyāti* = discernment, *puruṣa* = the primal self or consciousness itself, one of the two primary categories of Sāṁkhya-Yoga ontology. *guṇa* = quality, one's self is supposed to have the three *guṇa*-s of *sattva*, *rajaḥ* and *tamas*.
11. *samprajñāta* = conscious of objects, *vitarka* = debate on *sthūla* (coarse) objects, *vicāra* = reflection on *sūkṣma* (subtle) objects, *ānanda* = happiness/joy, *asmitā* = ego, feeling of personality.
12. *asamprajñāta* = not conscious of objects.
13. *saṁskāra* = subliminal impressions that *vṛtti*-s leave on the *citta*.
14. *prakṛti* = primary matter, one of the two primary categories in Sāṁkhya.

The other type (— *samprajñāta yoga* — is possible) through a precedence of respect, courage, *smṛti*, *samādhi* and *prajñā*.[15]

DEGREES OF SAMĀDHI (I.21-2)

21. तीव्रसंवेगानामत्यासन्नः।

tīvra-saṁvegānām-ati-āsannaḥ ।

For the keenly intense (*samādhi*) is very near.

22. मृदुमध्यधिमात्रत्वात्ततोऽपि विशेषः।

mṛdu-madhya-adhimātratvāt-tato'pi viśeṣaḥ ।

Because (this keenness) is gentle, moderate or extreme, there is (a *samādhi*) superior to this (near kind) also.

DISCUSSION ON ĪŚVARA[16] (I.23-8)

23. ईश्वरप्रणिधानाद्वा।

īśvara-praṇidhānād-vā ।

Or (*samādhi* is attained) by concentration on *īśvara*.

24. क्लेशकर्मविपाकाशयैरपरामृष्टाः पुरुषविशेष ईश्वरः

kleśa-karma-vipāka-āśayaiḥ-aparāmṛṣṭāḥ puruṣa-viśeṣa īśvaraḥ ।

Īśvara is a special type of *puruṣa*, untouched by *kleśa*, *karma*, *vipāka* or *āśaya*.[17]

---

15. *smṛti*= mindfulness (and not memory, as *smṛti* as memory is a *vṛtti*; see I.6 and I.11), *samādhi* = intense concentration, *prajñā* = insight.

16. *īśvara* = God, but here as I.24-6 shows, a special type of self or consciousness, a cognitive category. The presence of *īśvara* makes Yoga and Sāṁkhya distinct, as the latter is *nirīśvara*.

17. *karma* = one's doings in life, *vipāka* = fruition of *karma*-s, *āśaya* = latent deposits of *karma* for *kleśa*, see note 4.

25. तत्र निरतिशयं सर्वज्ञबीजम्।

tatra niratiśayaṁ sarvajña-bījam ।

In this (*īśvara*) is the seed of the omniscient at its best.

26. पूर्वेषामपि गुरुः कालेनानवच्छेदात्।

pūrveṣām-api guruḥ kālena-anavacchedāt ।

(*Īśvara* is) the *guru* of the primal ones (the sages) also, being unlimited by time.

27. तस्य वाचकः प्रणवः।

tasya vācakaḥ praṇavaḥ ।

The phonetic form expressing it (*īśvara*) is the *praṇava*.[18]

28. तज्जपस्तदर्थभावनम्।

tad-japas-tad-artha-bhāvanam ।

Its *japa*[19] and a reflection on its meaning (is to be made).

ANTARĀYA[20]-S AND THEIR ACCOMPANIMENTS (I.29-34)

29. ततः प्रत्यक्चेतनाधिगमोऽप्यन्तरायाभावश्च।

tataḥ pratyakcetanā-adhigamaḥ-api-antarāya-abhāvaḥ-ca ।

After this, right knowledge also needs *pratyakcetanā*[21] and a removal of *antarāya*-s.

30. व्याधिस्त्यानसंशयप्रमादालस्याविरतिभ्रान्तिदर्शनालब्धभूमिकत्वानवस्थितत्वानि चित्तविक्षेपास्तेऽन्तरायः।

vyādhi-styāna-saṁśaya-pramāda-ālasya-avirati-bhrāntidarśana-alabdhabhūmikatva-anavasthitatvāni citta-vikṣepa-aste'ntarāyaḥ ।

---

18. *praṇava* = the syllable *aum*, which has metaphysical connections.
19. *japa* = repetitive utterance.
20. *antarāya* = obstacle.
21. *pratyakcetanā* = introverted consciousness.

Sickness, langour, doubt, carelessness, laziness, non-cessation, wrong perception, not being able to attain ground (in some desired activity) and not being able to be situated (in that desired state) are the *vikṣepa*[22]-s of the *citta* which are *antarāya*-s.

31. दुःखदोर्मनस्याङगमेजयत्वश्वासप्रश्वास विक्षेपसहभूवः।

duḥkha-daurmanasya-aṅgamejayatva-śvāsa-praśvāsa vikṣepa-sahabhūvaḥ ।

Sadness, despondency, unsteadiness of the body and (irregular) inspiration and expiration are accompaniments of the *vikṣepa*-s.

32. तत्प्रतिषेधार्थमेकतत्त्वाभ्यासः।

tat-pratiṣedha-artham-ekatattva-abhyāsaḥ ।

To check them (one should perform) *abhyāsa* on a single entity.

33. मैत्रीकरुणामुदितोपेक्षाणां सुखदुःखपुण्यापुण्यविषयानां भावनातश्चित्तप्रसादनम्।

maitrī-karuṇā-muditā-upekṣāṇāṁ sukha-duḥkha-puṇya-apuṇya-viṣayānāṁ bhāvanātaḥ-citta-prasādanam ।

One can gain calm of the *citta* by a cultivation of friendliness towards happiness, compassion towards sorrow, joy towards merit and indifference towards demerit.

34. प्रच्छर्दनविधारणाभ्यां वा प्राणस्य।

pracchardana-vidhāraṇābhyāṁ vā prāṇasya ।

Or (one can do so) by a (regulated) expiration and retention of breath,

---

22. *vikṣepa* = distraction.

SUITABLE OBJECTS FOR ABHYĀSA (I.35-9)

35. विषयवती वा प्रवृत्तिरुत्पन्ना मनसः स्थितिनिबन्धनी।

viṣayavatī vā pravṛttiḥ-utpannā manasaḥ sthiti-nibandhanī ।

or (such a calm is possible when) a *pravṛtti* arises, connected to an object, bringing the *mana*[23] to stability.

36. विशोका वा ज्योतिष्मती।

viśokā vā jyotiṣmatī ।

(Such an object is) either without distress, and luminous,

37. वीतरागविषयं वा चित्तम।

vītarāgaviṣayaṁ vā cittam ।

or a *citta* without passion for (worldly) objects,

38. स्वप्ननिद्राज्ञानालम्बनं वा।

svapna-nidrā-jñāna-ālambanaṁ vā ।

or one based on knowledge attained through dream in sleep;

39. यथाभिमतध्यानाद्वा।

yathā-abhimata-dhyānād-vā ।

or (one can perform) *dhyāna*[24] on whatever one wishes.

POWER OF THE YOGĪ (I.40)

40. परमाणुपरममहत्त्वान्तोऽस्य वशीकारः

paramāṇu-paramamahattva-anto'sya vaśīkāraḥ ।

(The *yogī* can achieve) *vaśīkāra* from the smallest atom to the greatest magnitude.

---

23. *mana* = mind, like *citta*, one of the three elements of the *antaḥkaraṇa*. See Note 2, *pravṛtti* = propensities.
24. *dhyāna*= contemplation through concentration.

SAMĀPATTI[25] AND ITS TYPES (I.41-4)

41. क्षीणवृत्तेरभिजातस्येव मणेर्ग्रहितृग्रहणग्राह्येषु तत्स्थतदञ्जनता समापत्तिः।

kṣīṇa-vṛtteḥ-abhijātasya-iva maṇeḥ-grahitṛ-grahaṇa-grāhyeṣu tatstha-tadañjanatā samāpattiḥ ।

(When) on the *vṛtti*-s becoming dwindled, (the *citta*), like a gem's being coloured (by its background), takes the form of either the *grahitā*, or *grahaṇa* or the *grāhya*,[26] *samāpatti* (is said to have been achieved).

42. तत्र शब्दार्थज्ञानविकल्पैः सङ्कीर्णा सवितर्का समापत्तिः।

tatra śabda-artha-jñāna-vikalpaiḥ saṅkīrṇā savitarkā samāpattiḥ ।

Of these (all possible *samāpatti*-s), *savitarkā samāpatti*[27] is restricted by *vikalpa* constructions involving the word, intended object and the idea.

43. स्मृतिपरिशुद्धौ स्वरूपशूण्येवार्थमात्रनिर्भासा निर्वितर्का।

smṛti-pariśuddhau svarūpa-śūṇya-iva-arthamātra-nirbhāsā nirvitarkā ।

Once the *smṛti* is purified and emptied of its *svarūpa*, only the intended object gets illuminated, (and this *samāpatti*) is *nirvitarkā*.

44. एतयैव सविचारा निर्विचारा च सूक्ष्मविषया व्याख्याता।

etayaiva savicārā nirvicārā ca sūkṣmaviṣayā vyākhyātā ।

Similarly, (it can be) explained (how for) *sūkṣma* objects

---

25. *samāpatti* = the final stable stage in *yoga*.

26. *grahitā* = one who cognises, *grahaṇa* = the process/means of cognition, *grāhya* = that which is cognised.

27. *savitarkā* = with *vitarka*, similarly *nirvitarkā* (I.43) = without *vitarka*, for *vitarka*, see Note, 11. The feminine marker 'ā' is used at the end of these two adjectives because the noun they describe, '*samāpatti*' is feminine.

there are *savicārā* and *nirvicārā*[28] (*samāpatti*-s).

TWO TYPES OF SAMĀDHI (I.45-51)

45. **सूक्ष्मविषयत्वम् चालिङ्गपर्यवसानम्।**

sūkṣma-viṣayatvam ca-aliṅga-paryavasānam ।

Sūkṣma objects also terminate in *aliṅga*[29] (forms).

46. **ता एव सबीजः समाधिः।**

tā eva sabījaḥ samādhiḥ ।

These also (along with *nirvicārā samāpatti*) can cause *sabīja*[30] *samādhi*.

47. **निर्विचारवैशारद्येऽध्यात्मप्रसादः।**

nirvicāra-vaiśāradye'dhyātma-prasādaḥ ।

On clearness of the *nirvicāra* (*samāpatti*, one gets) internal calm.

48. **ऋतम्भरा तत्र प्रज्ञा।**

ṛtambharā tatra prajñā ।

In this (calm mind), *prajñā* is *ṛtambharā*.[31]

49. **श्रुतानुमानप्रज्ञाभ्यामन्यविषया विशेषार्थत्वात्।**

śruta-anumāna-prajñābhyām-anyaviṣayā viśeṣārthatvāt ।

(This *prajñā* is) different from the *prajñā* resulting from what is heard, or *anumāna*, in that it refers to particular objects.

---

28. *savicārā* = with *vicāra*; *nirvicāra* = without *vicāra*; for *vicāra*, see Note 11.

29. *aliṅga* = non-differentiable, without markers of differentiation.

30. *sabīja* = with 'seeds' (for further *vṛtti*-s); similarly *nirbīja* (I.51) = without seeds.

31. *ṛtambharā* = bearer of *ṛta*, *ṛta* is that frozen moment where immutable truth reveals itself.

50. तज्जः संस्कारोऽन्यसंस्कारप्रतिबन्धी।

tad-jaḥ saṁskāraḥ-anya-saṁskāra-pratibandhī ।

The *saṁskāra* arising from this hinders other *saṁskāra*-s.

51. तस्यापि निरोधे सर्वनिरोधन्निर्बीजः समाधिः।

tasya-api nirodhe sarva-nirodhaḥ-nirbījaḥ samādhiḥ ।

On *nirodha* of this (*saṁskāra*) also, all is *nirodha*-ed, (and) *nirbīja samādhi* (is attained).

BOOK TWO: *SĀDHANAPĀDA*
(On Means of Attainment)

KRIYĀ-YOGA[32] (II.1)

1. तपःस्वाध्यायेश्वरप्रणिधानानि क्रियायोगः।

tapaḥ-svādhyāya-īśvarapraṇidhānāni kriyāyogaḥ ।

Tapaḥ,[33] self-study and concentration on *īśvara* constitute *kriyā-yoga*.

TYPES OF KLEŚA AND MEANS FOR THEIR WEAKENING (II.2-11)

2. समाधिभावनार्थः क्लेशतनुकरणार्थश्च।

samādhi-bhāvanārthaḥ kleśa-tanu-karaṇārthaśca ।

(*Kriyā-yoga* is) for the cultivation of *samādhi* and the weakening of *kleśa*.

3. अविद्यास्मितारागद्वेषाभिनिवेशः क्लेशः।

avidyā-asmitā-rāga-dveṣa-abhiniveśaḥ kleśaḥ ।

Avidyā, *asmitā*, *rāga*, *dveṣa* and *abhiniveśa*[34] are the *kleśa*-s.

---

32. *kriyā-yoga* = The *yoga* of action.
33. *tapaḥ* = self-castigation.
34. *avidyā* = non-knowledge, *rāga* = passion, *dveṣa* = hatred, *abhiniveśa* = will to live, *asmitā* has already been explained in Note 11 to I.17.

4. अविद्या क्षेत्रमुत्तरेषां प्रसुप्ततनुविच्छिनोदाराणाम्।

avidyā kṣetram-uttareṣāṁ prasupta-tanu-vicchinna-udārāṇām ।

Avidyā is the field for the latter (four), whether they are dormant or weakened, dispersed or sustained.

5. अनित्याशुचिदुःखानात्मसु नित्यशुचिसुखात्मख्यातिरविद्या।

anitya-aśuci-duḥkha-anātmasu nitya-śuci-sukha-ātmakhyātiḥ-avidyā ।

Avidyā is the *khyāti* of *nitya*, purity, happiness and *ātmā* in what is *anitya*,[35] impure, sorrowful and not the *ātmā*.

6. दृग्दर्शनशक्त्योरेकात्मतेवास्मिता।

dṛk-darśana-śaktyoḥ-ekātmatā-iva-asmitā ।

When *dṛk-śakti* and *darśana-śakti*[36] appear to be one and the same, it is *asmitā*.

7. सुखानुशायी रागः।

sukha-anuśāyī rāgaḥ ।

Rāga is what bases itself in happiness.

8. दुःखानुशायी द्वेषः।

duḥkha-anuśāyī dveśaḥ ।

Dveṣa is what bases itself in sorrow.

9. स्वरसवाही विदुषोऽपि तथारूढोऽभिनिवेशः

svarasavāhī viduṣo'pi tathā-ārūḍhaḥ-abhiniveśaḥ ।

---

35. *nitya* = permanent, unchanging; *anitya* is just the opposite, *ātmā* = self. *Khyāti* has been explained in Note 10 to I.16.

36. *dṛkśakti* = the power of seeing, vision itself

darśanaśakti = the power by which one sees, one's own visual capacity.

Flowing on by its own *rasa*,[37] *abhiniveśa* boards even the wise ones.

10. ते प्रतिप्रसवहेयः सूक्ष्मः।

te pratiprasava-heyaḥ sūkṣmaḥ ।

When these (*kleśa*-s) are *sūkṣma*, they can be weakened through *pratiprasava.*[38]

11. ध्यानहेयस्तद्वृत्तयः।

dhyāna-heyaḥ-tad-vr̥ttayaḥ ।

The *vr̥tti*-s of these (*kleśa*-s) can be weakened through *dhyāna.*

ON KARMA (II.12-14)

12. क्लेशमूलः कर्माशयो दृष्टादृष्टजन्मवेदनीयः।

kleśa-mūlaḥ karma-āśayo dr̥ṣṭa-adr̥ṣṭa-janma-vedanīyaḥ ।

The *āśaya*-s of *karma* have their root in the *kleśa*-s and can be experienced in a birth so far seen or yet unseen.

13. सति मूले तद्विपाको जात्यायुर्भोगाः।

sati mūle tad-vipāko jāti-āyuḥ-bhogāḥ ।

As long as this root exists, there will be *vipāka* from it, realised through birth, length of life or *bhoga.*[39]

14. ते ह्लादपरितापफलः पुण्यापुण्यहेतुत्वात्।

te hlāda-paritāpa-phalaḥ puṇya-apuṇya-hetutvāt ।

These (*vipāka*-s) may result in intense joy or intense sorrow, depending on whether their causes are of merit or demerit.

---

37. *rasa* = essence; *rasa* has a more elaborate meaning in Indian poetics but it is beyond the scope of Yoga philosophy.

38. *pratiprasava* = inverse propagation.

39. *bhoga* = experience, acquisition, all other *karma*-related terms explained in Note 17 to I.24.

ON DUḤKHA (II.15-24)

15. परिणामतापसंस्कारदुःखैर्गुणवृत्तिविरोधाच्च दुःखमेव सर्वं विवेकिनः।

pariṇāma-tāpa-saṁskāra-duḥkhaiḥ-guṇa-vṛtti-virodhāñca duḥkhameva sarvaṁ vivekinaḥ ।

Duḥkha being *pariṇāma*, *tāpa* and *saṁskāra*-s (arising from) an opposition from the *vṛtti*-s of the *guṇa*-s too, all is *duḥkha* to the *vivekin*.[40]

16. हेयं दुःखमनागतम्।

heyaṁ duḥkham-anāgatam ।

That which is to be escaped is *duḥkha* yet to come.

17. द्रष्टृदृश्ययोः संयोगो हेयहेतुः

draṣṭṛ-dṛśyayoḥ saṁyogo heya-hetuḥ ।

The *saṁyoga*[41] between the seer and the object of sight is the reason for what is to be escaped.

18. प्रकाशक्रियास्थितिशीलं भूतेन्द्रियात्मकं भोगापवर्गार्थं दृश्यम।

prakāśa-kriyā-sthitiśīlaṁ bhūtendriya-ātmakaṁ bhoga-apavarga-arthaṁ-dṛśyam ।

The object of sight is that which has (a disposition to) brightness, action and inertia, has *bhūta* and the

---

40. *duḥkha* = pain, sorrow, since the discourse on *duḥkha* as a category begins here, it is from here that I retain *duḥkha* as a technical term. In all previous occurrences, it has been translated as 'sorrow'.

pariṇāma = mutation, *tāpa* = anxiety, *vivekin* = one with *viveka* or the discriminative faculty; one who can discriminate.

41. *saṁyoga* = conjunction. Here the term is used as a technical term for the conjunction between the *draṣṭā* (seer) and *dṛśya* (the object of sight). II.17-24 could have been classified as a discussion on *saṁyoga* but I prefer to include it within the broader discourse of *duḥkha* (II.15-24) because *saṁyoga* is shown as the cause for *duḥkha* and it is discussed here only because of this correlation.

indriya-s as its essence, and *bhoga* and *apavarga*[42] as its purpose.

19. विशेषाविशेषलिङ्गमात्रालिङ्गानि गुणपर्वाणि।

viśeṣa-aviśeṣa-liṅgamātra-aliṅgāni guṇa-parvāṇi ।

The divisions of the *guṇa*-s are *viśeṣa* and *aviśeṣa* — *liṅgamātra*[43] and *aliṅga* forms.

20. द्रष्टादृशिमात्रः शुद्धोऽपि प्रत्ययानुपश्यः।

draṣṭā-dṛśimātraḥ śuddho'pi pratyaya-anupaśyaḥ ।

The seer, who is nothing but the power of seeing, in spite of being undefiled, looks upon the presented idea.

21. तदर्थ एव दृश्यस्यात्मा।

tad-artha eva dṛśyasya-ātmā ।

The essence of the object of sight is for this purpose only.

22. कृतार्थं प्रति नष्टमप्यनष्टंतदन्यसाधारणत्वात्।

kṛta-arthaṁ prati naṣṭam-api-anaṣṭam-tad-anya-sādhāraṇatvāt ।

Though (the object of sight) ceases to be in one whose purpose has been accomplished, it itself does not get destroyed because of it being general to others.

23. स्वस्वामिशक्त्योः स्वरूपोपलब्धिहेतुः संयोगः।

sva-svāmi-śaktyoḥ svarūpa-upalabdhi-hetuḥ saṁyogaḥ ।

Saṁyoga is the reason behind the apperception of the nature of the powers of the properties and the proprietor.

---

42. *bhūta* = matter, *indriya* = bodily organs; there are ten *indriya*-s, five *karma-indriya*-s (the organs of action) and five *jñāna-indriya*-s (the sense-organs), *apavarga* = *mokṣa* or liberation.

43. *viśeṣa* = particular, *aviśeṣa* = non-particular, *liṅgamātra* = merely differentiable.

24. **तस्य हेतुरविद्या।**

tasya hetuḥ-avidyā ।

The reason for this (*saṁyoga*) is *avidyā*.

ON KAIVALYA[44] (II.25-7)

25. **तदभावात्संयोगाभावो हानं तद्दृशेः कैवल्यम्।**

tad-abhāvāt-saṁyoga-abhāvo hānaṁ tad-dṛśeḥ kaivalyam ।

When this (*duḥkha*) does not exist, *saṁyoga* does not exist, and this shows (one) the escape — *kaivalya*.

26. **विवेकख्यातिरविप्लवा हानोपायः।**

viveka-khyātiḥ-aviplavā hāna-upāyaḥ ।

The means for (this) escape is unwavering *viveka-khyāti*.[45]

27. **तस्य सप्तधा प्रान्तभूमिः प्रज्ञा।**

tasya saptadhā prāntabhūmiḥ prajñā ।

For him (there is) sevenfold *prajñā*, advancing towards the limits (of knowledge).

THE EIGHT AṄGA[46]-S OF YOGA (II.28-55)[47]

28. **योगाङ्गानुष्ठानातशुद्धिक्षये ज्ञानदीप्तिराविवेकख्यातेः।**

yoga-aṅga-anuṣṭhānāt-aśuddhi-kṣaye jñāna-dīptiḥ-āvivekakhyāteḥ ।

---

44. *kaivalya* = (lit. meaning) isolation; the *yoga* word for *mokṣa* = liberation.

45. *viveka-khyāti* = discriminative discernment. For *viveka* see Note 40 on II.15 and for *khyāti* see Note 10. on I.16.

46. *aṅga* = organ/limb.

47. That is to the end of Book II. Actually only the first five *aṅga*-s get discussed in Book II. The remaining three are discussed in Book III, *sūtra*-s 1-3.

Once the *aṅga*-s of *yoga* are performed, impurities get dwindled and an illumination of knowledge appears, leading to *viveka-khyāti*.

29. यमनियमासनप्राणायामप्रत्याहारधारणाध्यानसमाधयोऽष्टावङ्गानि।

yama-niyama-āsana-prāṇāyāma-pratyāhāra-dhāraṇā-dhyāna-samādhayaḥ-aṣṭo-aṅgāni ।

yama, *niyama*, *āsana*, *prāṇāyāma*, *pratyāhāra*, *dhāraṇā*,[48] *dhyāna* and *samādhi* are the eight *aṅga*-s.

30. अहिंसासत्यास्तेयब्रह्मचर्यापरिग्रहा यमाः।

ahiṁsā-satya-asteya-brahmacarya-aparigrahā yamāḥ ।

Abstinence from violence, falsehood, theft, incontinence and acquisition are the (five) *yama*-s.

31. जातिदेशकालसमयानवछिन्नाः सार्वभौमाः महाव्रतम्।

jāti-deśa-kāla-samaya-anavachinnāḥ sārvabhaumāḥ mahāvratam ।

When these (*yama*-s) are unhindered by class, place, period or time, they constitute a sovereign *mahāvrata*.[49]

32. शौचसन्तोषतपःस्वाध्यायेश्वरप्रणिधानानि नियमः।

śauca-santoṣa-tapaḥ-svādhyāya-īśvarapraṇidhānāni niyamaḥ ।

Cleanliness, contentment, *tapaḥ*, self-study and concentration on *īśvara* are the (five) *niyama*-s.

33. वितर्कबाधने प्रतिपक्षभावनम्।

vitarka-bādhane pratipakṣa-bhāvanam ।

If *vitarka* produces hindrances, its opposites should be cultivated.

---

48. *yama* = abstention, *niyama* = observance, *āsana* = posture, *prāṇāyāma* = regulated control of breath, *pratyāhāra* = withdrawal (of the senses), *dhāraṇā* = forming of idea.

49. *mahāvrata* = great course of conduct.

34. वितर्का हिंसादयः कृतकारितानुमोदिता लोभक्रोधमोहपूर्वका। मृदुमध्याधिमात्रा दुःखाज्ञानानन्तफला इति प्रतिपक्षभावनम्।।

vitarkā hiṁsā-ādayaḥ kṛta-kārita-anumoditā lobha-krodha-moha-pūrvakā ।
mṛdu-madhya-adhimātrā duḥkha-ajñāna-anantaphalā iti pratipakṣa-bhāvanam ।।

Since (modes of) *vitarka*, like violence, etc., whether be done, caused to be done, or approved to be done, whether preceded by greed, anger or infatuation, whether gentle, moderate or extreme, always ends in *duḥkha* and lack of knowledge, its opposites should be cultivated.

35. अहिंसाप्रतिष्ठायां तत्सन्निधौ वैरत्यागः।

ahiṁsā-pratiṣṭhāyāṁ tat-sannidhau vaira-tyāgaḥ ।

On the establishment of abstinence from violence, one gets associated with a giving up of enmity.

36. सत्यप्रतिष्ठायां क्रियाफलाश्रयत्वम्।

satya-pratiṣṭhāyāṁ kriyā-phala-āśrayatvam ।

On the establishment of abstinence from falsehood, actions and their consequences get rooted (in one).

37. अस्तेयप्रतिष्ठायां सर्वरत्नोपस्थानम्।

asteya-pratiṣṭhāyāṁ sarva-ratna-upasthānam ।

On the establishment of abstinence from theft, all jewels present themselves.

38. ब्रह्मचर्यप्रतिष्ठायां वीर्यलाभः।

brahmacarya-pratiṣṭhāyāṁ vīrya-lābhaḥ ।

On the establishment of abstinence from incontinence, one gains courage (or sexual powers, *vīrya* also meaning semen).

39. अपरिग्रहस्थैर्ये जन्मकथन्तासम्बोधः।

aparigraha-sthairye janma-kathantā-sambodhaḥ ।

On stability in abstinence from acquisition (one gains) through knowledge of the conditions of birth.

40. शौचात्स्वाङ्गजुगुप्सा परैरसंसर्गः।

śaucāt-sva-aṅga-jugupsā paraiḥ-asaṁsargaḥ ।

Cleanliness develops disgust for one's own body, leading to lack of intercourse with others.

41. सत्वशुद्धिसौमनस्यैकाग्र्येन्द्रियजयात्मदर्शनयोग्यत्वानि च

satva-śuddhi-saumanasya-aikāgrya-indriyajaya-ātmadarśana-yogyatvāni ca ।

(Clealiness also leads to) purity of the *satva* (of the self), gentleness, singleness of intent, subjugation of the *indriya*-s and fitness for *ātmadarśana*.[50]

42. सन्तोषादनुत्तमसुखलाभः।

santoṣāt-anuttama-sukha-lābhaḥ ।

Through contentment, one gains unsurpassed joy.

43. कायेन्द्रियसिद्धिरशुद्धिक्षयात्तपसः

kāya-indriya-siddhiḥ-aśuddhi-kṣayāt-tapasaḥ ।

Tapaḥ leads to a purification of the body and the *indriya*-s through a dwindling away of impurities.

44. स्वाध्यायादिष्टदेवतासम्प्रयोगः।

svādhyāyāt-iṣṭadevatā-samprayogaḥ ।

Through self-study there is a communion with one's chosen deity.

---

50. *ātmadarśana* = a sight of the *ātmā*, one's self, *satva* = thatness; the essence of an entity phenomenal.

45. समाधिसिद्धिरीश्वरप्रणिधानात्।

samādhi-siddhiḥ-īśvara-praṇidhānāt ।

There is a perfection in *samādhi* through concentration on *īśvara*.

46. स्थिरसुखमासनम्।

sthira-sukham-āsanam ।

Āsana is a stable and easy (posture).

47. प्रयत्नशैथिल्यानन्तसमापत्तिभ्याम्।

prayatna-śaithilya-ananta-samāpattibhyām ।

(*Āsana* is possible) by a relaxation of efforts or a *samāpatti* on what is *ananta*.[51]

48. ततः द्वन्द्वानभिघातः।

tataḥ dvandva-anabhighātaḥ ।

Thereafter, (such a one who has performed *āsana*-s) is unharmed by *dvandva*.[52]

49. तस्मिन् सति श्वासप्रश्वासयोर्गतिविच्छेदः प्राणायामः।

tasmin sati śvāsa-praśvāsayoḥ-gati-vicchedaḥ prāṇāyāmaḥ ।

Following this (*āsana*) comes the cutting-off of the flow of inspiration and expiration, (which is) *prāṇāyāma*.

50. बाध्याभ्यन्तरस्तम्भवृत्तिर्देशकालसङ्ख्याभिः परिदृष्टो दीर्घसूक्ष्म।

bāhya-abhyantara-stambha-vṛttiḥ-deśa-kāla-saṁkhyābhiḥ paridṛṣṭo dīrgha-sūkṣma ।

The *vṛtti* of (breathing being about) external, internal and withheld (air, its regulation according to) space, time

---

51. *ananta* = endless, whatever is immutable, normally refers to god.
52. *dvandva* = turmoil, here mostly mental rather than physical violence.

and number, gets seen in the protracted and *sūkṣma* (process of *prāṇāyāma*).

51. बाह्याभ्यन्तरविषयाक्षेपी चतुर्थः।

bāhya-abhyantara-viṣaya-akṣepī caturthaḥ ।

The relative relationship between external and internal substance (i.e., air) is determined by the rule of fourths.[53]

52. ततः क्षीयते प्रकाशावरणम्।

tataḥ kṣīyate prakāśa-āvaraṇam ।

Thereafter, the covering, that veils illumination, dwindles.

53. धारणासु च योग्यता मनसः।

dhāraṇāsu ca yogyatā manasaḥ ।

And from *dhāraṇā* arises competence of the *mana*.

54. स्वविषयासम्प्रयोगे चित्तस्वरूपानुकार इवेन्द्रियानां प्रत्याहारः।

sva-viṣaya-asamprayoge citta-svarūpa-anukāra iva-indriyānāṁ pratyāhāraḥ ।

Pratyāhāra is an imitation by the *citta* of its *svarūpa*, as also through the *indriya*-s, by disjoining them from their objects of perception.

55. ततः परमा वश्यतेन्द्रियाणाम्।

tataḥ paramā vaśyatā-indriyāṇām ।

After this (*pratyāhāra*), there is a complete *vaśīkāra* over the *indriya*-s.

---

53. The three stages of *prāṇāyāma*, *pūraka* or inspiration, *recaka* or expiration and *kumbhaka* or withholding breath, are regulated by a simple rule of fourths, so that if one inhales for one unit of time, one has to withhold the breath for four units and exhale it over a period of two units.

BOOK THREE: *VIBHŪTIPĀDA*
(On the Powers Attained)

THE REMAINING THREE AṄGA-S (III.1-3)

1. **देशबन्धश्चित्तस्य धारणा।**

   deśa-bandhaḥ-cittasya dhāraṇā ।

   Binding the *citta* to one place is *dhāraṇā*.

2. **तत्र प्रत्ययैकतानता ध्यानम्।**

   tatra pratyaya-ekatānatā dhyānam ।

   Focusing the end of this (*dhāraṇā*) is *dhyāna*.

3. **तदेवार्थमात्रनिर्भासंस्वरूपशूण्यमिवसमाधिः।**

   tadeva-arthamātra-nirbhāsaṁ-svarūpa-śūṇyam-iva-samādhiḥ ।

   Samādhi is when this (*dhyāna*) shines forth into only the intended object, (the sign thereby having) purged itself of its *svarūpa*.

SAṀYAMA[54] AS LEADING TO NIRBĪJA SAMĀDHI (III.4-10)

4. **त्रयमेकत्र संयमः।**

   trayam-ekatra saṁyamaḥ ।

   The three (*dhāraṇā*, *dhyāna*, *samādhi*) have to be *saṁyama*-ed simultaneously.

5. **तज्जयात्प्रज्ञालोकः।**

   tad-jayāt-prajñā-ālokaḥ ।

   Victory over this (*saṁyama*) leads to the light of *prajñā*.

6. **तस्य भूमिषु विनियोगः।**

   tasya bhūmiṣu viniyogaḥ ।

---

54. *saṁyama* = control.

The applicability of this (*prajñā*) is to the base (of all cognition, i.e., the *citta*).

7. त्रयमन्तरङ्गं पूर्वेभ्यः।

trayam-antaraṅgaṁ pūrvebhyaḥ

These three (*aṅga*-s) are more intrinsic than the earlier (five).

8. तदपि बहिरङ्ग निर्बीजस्य।

tad-api bahiraṅga nirbījasya।

(But) even these (three) are extrinsic to *nirbīja* (*samādhi*).

9. व्युत्थाननिरोधसंस्कारयोरभिभावप्रादुर्भावौनिरोधक्षणचित्तान्वयो निरोधपरिणामः।

vyutthāna-nirodha-saṁskārayoḥ-abhibhāva-prādurbhāvau-nirodha-kṣaṇa-citta-anvayo nirodha-pariṇāmaḥ।

The synthesis in the *citta* of the becoming invisible of the *saṁskāra*-s of *vyutthāna*[55] and the becoming visible of those of *nirodha*, at the time of *nirodha*, is the *pariṇāma* of *nirodha*.

10. तस्य प्रशान्तवाहिता संस्कारात्।

tasya praśāntavāhitā saṁskārāt।

In that (*citta*) the *saṁskāra*-s flow peacefully.

PARIṆĀMA AND ITS SAṀYAMA (III.11-16)

11. सर्वार्थतैकाग्रतयोः क्षयोदयौ चित्तस्यसमाधिपरिणामः।

sarva-arthatā-ekāgratayoḥ kṣaya-udayau cittasya-samādhi-pariṇāmaḥ।

The dwindling of thought about all objects and the uprisal of singleness of intent in the *citta* is the *pariṇāma* of *samādhi*.

---

55. *vyutthāna* = uprising.

12. ततः पुनः शान्तोदितौ तुल्यप्रत्ययौ चित्तस्यैकाग्रतापरिणामः।

tataḥ punaḥ śānta-uditau tulya-pratyayau cittasya-ekāgratā-pariṇāmaḥ ।

Again when the quiescent and the uprisen states (thus presented) become similar, it is the *pariṇāma* of singleness of intent of the *citta*.

13. एतेन भूतेन्द्रियेषु धर्मलक्षणावस्थापरिणामा व्याख्याताः।

etena bhūta-indriyeṣu dharma-lakṣaṇa-avasthā-pariṇāmā vyākhyātā ।

Similarly for the *bhūta* and the *indriya*-s, *pariṇāma* can be of three types — *dharma*, *lakṣaṇa* and *avasthā*[56] *pariṇāma*-s.

14. शान्तोदिताव्यपदेश्यधर्मानुपाती धर्मी।

śānta-udita-avyapadeśya-dharma-anupātī dharmī ।

A substance which conforms to quiescent, uprisen or indeterminable *dharma* is known as *dharmī*.

15. क्रमान्यत्वं परिणामान्यत्वे हेतुः।

krama-anyatvaṁ pariṇāma-anyatve hetuḥ ।

The difference in sequence is the reason for the difference in *pariṇāma*-s.

16. परिणामत्रयसंयमादतीतानागतज्ञानम्।

pariṇāma-traya-saṁyamāt-atīta-anāgata-jñānam ।

A *saṁyama* on the three types of *pariṇāma* (those based on *dharma*, *lakṣaṇa* and *avasthā*) brings in knowledge of the past and future.

OTHER SAṀYAMA-S AND POWERS ATTAINED THEREFROM (III.17-52)

17. शब्दार्थप्रत्ययानामितरेतराध्यासात् सङ्करस्तत्प्रविभागसंयमात् सर्वभूतरुतज्ञानम्।

---

56. *dharma* = intrinsic properties, *lakṣaṇa* = manifest properties, *avasthā* = current condition.

śabda-artha-pratyayānām-itaretara-adhyāsāt saṅkaraḥ-tat-pravibhāga-saṁyamāt sarva-bhūtaruta-jñānam ।

Word, intended object and idea are confused to be one and the same. Through a *saṁyama* on their differences (one gains) knowledge of the cries of all living beings.

18. **संस्कारसाक्षात्करणात् पूर्वजातिज्ञानम्।**

saṁskāra-sākṣātkaraṇāt pūrva-jāti-jñānam ।

As a result of direct perception of one's *saṁskāra*-s there is knowledge of earlier births.

19. **प्रत्ययस्य परचित्तज्ञानम्।**

pratyayasya paracitta-jñānam ।

(Because of *saṁyama*) of the presented idea there is knowledge about other *citta*-s.

20. **न च तत्सालम्बनं तस्याविषयीभूतत्वात्।**

na ca tat-sālambanaṁ tasya-aviṣayī-bhūtatvāt ।

But this knowledge is not with a proper base as it is not a subject of (the *yogī*'s *citta*).

21. **कायरूपसंयमात् तद्ग्राह्यशक्तिस्तम्भे चक्षुप्रकाशासम्प्रयोगेऽन्तर्धानम्।**

kāya-rūpa-saṁyamāt tad-grāhya-śakti-stambhe cakṣu-prakāśa-asamprayogeḥ-antardhānam ।

When there is a *saṁyama* on the (outer) form of the body, its power to be *grāhya* gets withheld, and the resulting disjunction between the faculty of vision and light, (the *yogī* can achieve) *antardhāna*.[57]

22. **सोपक्रमं निरुपक्रमं च कर्म तत्संयमातपरान्तज्ञानमरिष्टेभ्यो वा।**

sa-upakramaṁ nirupakramaṁ ca karma tat-saṁyamāt-aparānta-jñānam-ariṣṭebhyo vā ।

57. *antardhāna* = to vanish, to become indiscernible.

Karma is of two types — with and without progress. *Saṁyama* on this (two-fold *karma*) or on *ariṣṭa*[58] produces knowledge of the other end (of life, i.e., death).

23. मैत्र्यादिषु बलानि।

maitrī-ādiṣu balāni ।

From (*saṁyama* on) friendliness, etc., come the *bala*-s.[59]

24. बलेषु हस्तिबलादीनि।

baleṣu hasti-balādīni ।

From the *bala*-s, one can become as strong as elephants, etc.

25. प्रवृत्त्यालोकन्यासात् सूक्ष्मव्यवहितविप्रकृष्टज्ञानम्।

pravṛtti-āloka-nyāsāt sūkṣma-vyavahita-viprakṛṣṭa-jñānam ।

As a result of casting the light of a *pravṛtti*, (arises) the knowledge of *sūkṣma*, far off and obscure objects.

26. भूवनज्ञानं सूर्ये संयमात्।

bhūvana-jñānaṁ sūrye saṁyamāt ।

As a result of *saṁyama* on the sun, (there is) knowledge of the whole universe.

27. चन्द्रे ताराव्यूहज्ञानम्

candre tārā-vyūha-jñānam ।

(Through *saṁyama*) on the moon, (one gets) the knowledge of the arrangement of stars.

28. ध्रुवे तदगतिज्ञानम्

dhruve tadgati-jñānam ।

---

58. *ariṣṭa* = signs of death.

59. *bala* = strength.

(Through *saṁyama*) on the pole-star (one gets) knowledge of the movement of stars.

29. नाभिचक्रे कायव्यूहज्ञानम्।

nābhi-cakre kāya-vyūha-jñānam ।

(Through *saṁyama*) on the umbilical circle, (one gets) knowledge of the arrangement of the body.

30. कण्ठकूपे क्षुत्पिपासानिवृत्तिः।

kaṇṭhakūpe kṣut-pipāsā-nivṛttiḥ ।

(*Saṁyama*) on the laryngo-oesophagal tract is followed by a cessation of hunger and thirst.

31. कूर्मनाड्यां स्थैर्यम्।

kūrma-nāḍyāṁ sthairyam ।

(*Saṁyama*) on the *kūrma-nāḍī*[60] (leads to) motionlessness.

32. मूर्धाज्योतिषि सिद्धदर्शनम्।

mūrdhā-jyotiṣi siddha-darśanam ।

(*Saṁyama*) on the *mūrdhā-jyoti* (leads to) *siddha-darśana*.[61]

33. प्रतिभाद्वासर्वम।

pratibhāt-vā-sarvam ।

Or as a result of *pratibhā*,[62] all (knowledge is attained).

34. हृदये चित्तसंवित्।

hṛdaye citta-saṁvit ।

---

60. *kūrma-nāḍī* = a tortoise-shaped tube just beneath the laryngo-oesophagal tract.

61. *siddha-darśana* = sight of the state of *siddhi* (fulfilment) *mūrdhā-jyoti* = cranial radiance, radiance from the *suṣumnā-nāḍī*.

62. *pratibhā* = (lit.) inner radiance — talent.

(*Saṁyama*) on the heart (leads to) consciousness of the *citta*.

35. सत्वपुरुषयोरत्यन्तासङ्कीर्णयोः प्रत्ययाविशेषो भोगः परार्थात्स्वार्थ-संयमात्पुरुषज्ञानम्।

satva-puruṣayoḥ-atyanta-asaṁkīrṇayoḥ pratyaya-aviśeṣo bhogaḥ prarārthāt-svārtha-saṁyamāt-puruṣa-jñānam ।

The perception of the very distinct *satva* and *puruṣa* as the same is *bhoga*. A *saṁyama* on the intrinsic object of these two very different objects (leads to) knowledge of *puruṣa*.

36. ततः प्रातिभश्रावणवेदनादर्शास्वादवार्त्ता जायन्ते।

tataḥ prātibha-śrāvaṇa-vedanā-ādarśa-āsvāda-vārtā jāyante ।

From this arises the *pratibhā* leading to the (supernal) faculties of hearing, touch, sight, taste and smell.

37. ते समाधावुपसर्गा व्युत्थाने सिद्धयः।

te samādhau-upasargā vyutthāne siddhayaḥ ।

In *samādhi*, these (supernal senses) are *upasarga*-s,[63] but in *vyutthāna*, they are *siddhi*-s.

38. बन्धकारणशैथिल्यात्प्रचारसंवेदनाच्च चित्तस्य परशरीरावेशः।

bandha-kāraṇa-śaithilyāt-pracāra-saṁvedanāt-ca cittasya-paraśarīra-āveśaḥ ।

As a result of slackening the causes of bondage, and an understanding of the (process of the *citta*'s) proliferation, the *citta* penetrates another body.

39. उदानजयाज्जलपङ्ककण्टकादिष्वसङ्ग उत्क्रान्तिश्च।

udāna-jayāt-jala-paṅka-kaṇṭaka-ādiṣu-asaṅga utkrāntiḥ-ca ।

---

63. *upasarga* = symptoms of obstacles.

As a result of mastery over *udāna*,[64] there is no adhesion to water, mud, thorns, etc., and (one gains an) upward movement.

40. **समानजयाज्ज्वलनम्।**

samāna-jayāt-jvalanam ।

As a result of mastery over *samāna*[65] (the *yogī* gains) an incandescence.

41. **श्रोत्राकाशयोः सम्बन्धसंयमाद् दिव्यं श्रोत्रम्।**

śrotra-ākāśayoḥ sambandha-saṁyamād divyaṁ śrotram ।

As a result of *saṁyama* upon the relation between the organ of hearing and air, (one gains) the supernal organ of hearing.

42. **कायाकाशयोः सम्बन्धसंयमाल्लघुतूलसमापत्तेश्चाकाशगमनम्।**

kāya-ākāśayoḥ sambandha-saṁyamāt-laghu-tūla-samāpatteḥ-ca-ākāśa-gamanam ।

As a result of *saṁyama* upon the relation between the body and air, and through the *samāpatti* of lightness, as in cotton, (one gains the power of) movement through air.

43. **बहिरकल्पिता वृत्तिर्महाविदेहा ततः प्रकाशावरणक्षयः।**

bahiḥ-akalpitā vṛttiḥ-mahāvidehā tataḥ prakāśa-āvaraṇa-kṣaya ।

An external unplanned *vṛtti* is the *mahāvideha*.[66] From it (arises) a dwindling of the covering that veils illumination.

---

64. *udāna* = the movement of bodily fluids from throat upwards.
65. *samāna* = the movement of bodily fluids, mostly digestive ones, that operate between the heart and the navel.
66. *mahāvideha* = the great discarnate one.

44. स्थूलस्वरूपसूक्ष्मान्वयार्थवत्वसंयमाद् भूतजयः।

sthūla-svarūpa-sūkṣma-anvaya-arthavatva-saṁyamād bhūta-jayaḥ ।

As a result of *saṁyama* over the *svarūpa* of *sthūla* objects and the objectiveness of the inherence of *sūkṣma* objects, (one gains) mastery over the *bhūta*.

45. ततोऽणिमादिप्रादुर्भावः कायसम्पत्तद्धर्मानभिघातश्च।

tatoḥ-aṇimā-ādi-prādurbhāvaḥ kāya-sampat-tad-dharma-anabhighātaḥ-ca ।

This (*bhūta-jaya*) leads to the coming of (the eight *siddhi*-s like) *aṇimā*,[67] etc., resulting in a perfection of the body, it receiving no obstruction from its *dharma*-s.

46. रूपलावण्यबलवज्रसंहननत्वानि कायसम्पत्।

rūpa-lāvaṇya-bala-vajra-saṁhananatvāni kāya-sampat ।

Beauty, grace, *bala* and the strength of a thunderbolt are the perfections of the body.

47. ग्रहणस्वरूपास्मितान्वयार्थवत्वसंयमादिन्द्रियजयः

grahaṇa-svarūpa-asmitā-anvaya-arthavatva-saṁyamāt-indriya-jayaḥ ।

As a result of *saṁyama* over *grahaṇa*, *svarūpa*, *asmitā*, inherence and objectiveness, (one gains) mastery over the *indriya*-s.

48. ततो मनोजवित्वं विकरणभावः प्रधानजयश्च।

tato manoja-vitvaṁ vikaraṇa-bhāvaḥ pradhāna-jayaḥ-ca ।

This results in a speed in the *mana*, gaining of knowledge disjunct from the body, and a mastery over the

---

67. *aṇimā* = the state of an *aṇu* (atom), atomisation; one of the eight *siddhi*-s.

pradhāna.[68]

49. सत्वपुरुषान्यताख्यातिमात्रस्य सर्वभावाधिष्ठातृत्वं सर्वज्ञातृत्वं च।

satva-puruṣa-anyatā-khyāti-mātrasya sarva-bhāva-adhiṣṭhātṛtvaṁ sarvajñātṛtvaṁ ca ।

From a *khyāti* of the difference between *satva* and *puruṣa* arises (one's) being situated in all states of existence and knowing all.

50. तदवैराग्यादपि दोषबीजक्षये कैवल्यम्।

tad-vairāgyāt-api doṣabījakṣaye kaivalyam ।

On *vairāgya* (for these also, the seed of *doṣa*[69] dwindles, leading to *kaivalya*.

51. स्थान्युपनिमन्त्रणे सङ्गस्मयाकरणं पुनरनिष्टप्रसङ्गात्।

sthānī-upanimantraṇe saṅga-asmaya-akaraṇaṁ punaḥ-aniṣṭa-prasaṅgāt ।

On being invited by people of stature, one should neither cohabit with them, nor show any pride, (because) *aniṣṭa*[70] may recur from it.

52. क्षणतत्क्रमयोः संयमाद्विवेकजं ज्ञानम्।

kṣaṇa-tat-kramayoḥ saṁyamāt-vivekajaṁ jñānam ।

As a result of *saṁyama* on moments and their sequence, (one attains) knowledge arising from the *viveka*.

CULMINATION OF SAMĀDHI IN KAIVALYA (III.53-5)

53. जातिलक्षणदेशैरन्यतानवच्छेदात्तुल्ययोस्ततः प्रतिपत्तिः।

jāti-lakṣaṇa-deśaiḥ-anyatā-anavacchedāt-tulyayoḥ-tataḥ pratipattiḥ ।

---

68. *pradhāna* = (lit.) principal — the principal cause, another name for *prakṛti*.

69. *doṣa* = fault.

70. *aniṣṭa* = harm, some harmful hindrance.

From this (knowledge from the *viveka*) arises the deeper knowledge of (two) comparable things (*satva* and *puruṣa*), which cannot be distinguished in terms of class, *lakṣaṇa*, or space.

54. तारकं सर्वविषयं सर्वथाविषयमक्रमं चेति विवेकजं ज्ञानम्।

tārakaṁ sarva-viṣayaṁ sarvathā-viṣayam-akramaṁ ca-iti vivekajaṁ jñānam ।

The knowledge from the *viveka* is a deliverer that has all things and all times as its object, and is itself without sequence.

55. सत्वपुरुषयोः शुद्धिसाम्ये कैवल्यम्।

satva-puruṣayoḥ śuddhi-sāmye kaivalyam ।

When the purity of *satva* and *puruṣa* are of the same degree, *kaivalya* is achieved.

BOOK FOUR: *KAIVALYAPĀDA*
(On Isolation)

SUBSTANCES AND VĀSANĀ[71] (IV.1-13)

1. जन्मौषधिमन्त्रतपः समाधिजाः सिद्धयः।

janma-oṣadhi-mantra-tapaḥ samādhi-jāḥ siddhayaḥ ।

Siddhi-s proceed from birth, drugs, incantatory spell, *tapaḥ* or *samādhi*.

2. जात्यन्तरपरिणामः प्रकृत्यापुरात्।

jāti-antara-pariṇāmaḥ prakṛti-āpurāt ।

The *pariṇāma* into another birth is (because of) the filling-in of *prakṛti*.

3. निमित्तमप्रयोजकं प्रकृतीनां वरणभेदस्तु ततः क्षेत्रिकवत्।

---

71. *vāsanā* = desire, subconscious impressions.

nimittam-aprayojakaṁ prakṛtīnāṁ varaṇa-bhedastu tataḥ kṣetrikavat ।

The *nimitta*[72] gives no impulse to the *prakṛti*, but cuts the barrier to that (*prakṛti*), like a peasant (ploughing his field).

4. निर्माणचित्तान्यस्मितामात्रात्।

nirmāṇa-cittāni-asmitā-mātrāt ।

Creation of *citta*-s (may arise) from *asmitā* alone.

5. प्रवृत्तिभेदे प्रयोजकं चित्तमेकमनेकेषाम्।

pravṛtti-bhede prayojakaṁ cittam-ekam-anekeṣām ।

Though there is a variety of *pravṛtti*-s, the *citta*, which necessitates the many, is one.

6. तत्र ध्यानजमनाशयम्।

tatra dhyānajam-anāśayam ।

Of these (five types of *siddhi*-s) the one proceeding from *dhyāna* (i.e., from *tapaḥ* and *samādhi*) leaves no *āśaya*.

7. कर्माशुक्लाकृष्णं योगिनस्त्रिविधमितरेषाम्।

karma-aśukla-akṛṣṇaṁ yoginaḥ-trividham-itareṣām ।

Karma is neither white nor black for *yogī*-s, while for others it may be of three types (white, black, and both black and white).

8. ततस्तद्विपाकानुगुणानामेवाभिव्यक्तिर्वासनानाम्।

tataḥ-tad-vipāka-anuguṇānām-eva-abhivyaktiḥ-vāsanānām ।

From these (three types of *karma*) what get manifest

---

72. *nimitta* = the effective cause, as opposed to *prakṛti* which is the evolving cause. Both *prakṛti* and *nimitta* are, however, *kāraṇa* or cause.

are the *vāsanā*-s only which correspond to the *vipāka*-s (of the *karma*).

9. जातिदेशकालव्यवहितानामप्यनन्तर्यं स्मृतिसंस्कारयोरेकरूपत्वात्।

jāti-deśa-kāla-vyavahitānām-api-anantarya smṛti-saṁskārayoḥ-ekarūpatvāt।

Though (the *vāsanā*-s) are differentiated in class, space and time, there is a non-differentiation because of the correspondence between *smṛti* and the *saṁskāra*-s.

10. तासामनादित्वां चाशिषो नित्यत्वात्।

tāsām-anāditvāṁ ca-āśiṣo nityatvāt।

Moreover, (*vāsanā*-s are) *anādi*,[73] since desire is *nitya*.

11. हेतुफलाश्रयालम्बनैः सङ्गृहीतात्वातेषामभावे तदभावः।

hetu-phala-āśraya-ālambanaiḥ saṁgṛhītātvāt-eṣām-abhāve tad-abhāvaḥ।

As a result of (*vāsanā*-s) being collected from cause, result, the substratum and stimulus, if these cease to exist, so do these (*vāsanā*-s).

12. अतीतानागतं स्वरूपतोऽस्त्यध्वभेदाद्धर्माणाम्।

atīta-anāgataṁ svarūpataḥ-asti-adhvabhedāt-dharmāṇām।

The *svarūpa* (of *vāsanā*-s) exists in past and future too as temporal forms of their *dharma*-s.

13. तेव्यक्तसूक्ष्मा गुणात्मानः।

te-vyakta-sūkṣmā guṇātmānaḥ।

These (*dharma*-s of *vāsanā*-s as manifest in their three temporal forms) are either *vyakta*[74] or *sūkṣma*, and their *ātmā* is the *guṇa*-s.

---

73. *anādi* = without a beginning, one whose beginning is not known.

74. *vyakta* = in the phenomenalised form.

COGNITION OF VASTU AND THE CITI[75] (IV.14-23)

14. परिणामैकत्वाद् वस्तुतत्वम्।

pariṇāma-ekatvād vastu-tatvam ।

The 'thatness' of a *vastu* is because of a singleness of *pariṇāma*,

15. वस्तुसाम्ये चित्तभेदात्तयोर्विभक्तः पन्थाः।

vastu-sāmye citta-bhedāt-tayoḥ-vibhaktaḥ panthāḥ ।

(and not because of its cognition as) a *vastu* being one but *citta*-s being varied, (the two) are on two different planes of existence.

16. न चैकचित्ततन्त्रं वस्तु तदप्रमाणकं तदा किं स्यात्।

na ca-eka-citta-tantraṁ vastu tad-apramāṇakaṁ tadā kiṁ syāt ।

A *vastu* is not dependent on a single *citta* (because then in certain cases) it cannot be provided a *pramāṇa* for (by that *citta*), and then what will it be?

17. तदुपरागापेक्षित्वाच्चित्तस्य वस्तु ज्ञाताज्ञातम्।

tad-uparāga-apekṣitvāt-cittasya vastu jñāta-ajñātam ।

A *vastu* is known or not known by virtue of its affecting (or not-affecting) the *citta*.

18. सदा ज्ञातश्चित्तवृत्तयस्तत्प्रभो पुरुषस्यापरिणामित्वात्।

sadā jñātaḥ-citta-vṛttayaḥ-tat-prabhoḥ puruṣasya-apariṇāmitvāt ।

A master of that (*citta*) always knows his *citta-vṛtti*-s and thus for him the *puruṣa* has no *pariṇāma*.

19. न तत्स्वाभासं दृश्येत्वात्।

na tat-sva-ābhāsaṁ dṛśyetvāt ।

---

75. *vastu* = thing, object, *citi* = intellect, the intentional cognising agency.

That (*citta*) does not illumine itself, being the object for sight,

20. एकसमये चोभयानवधारणम्।

eka-samaye ca-ubhaya-anavadhāraṇam ।

as there cannot be a cognition of both (the subject and object of sight) at the same time.

21. चित्तान्तरदृश्ये बुद्धिबुद्धेरतिप्रसङ्गः स्मृतिसङ्करश्च।

citta-antara-dṛśye buddhi-buddheḥ-atiprasaṅgaḥ smṛti-saṅkaraḥ-ca ।

If one *citta* was the object for sight for another, there would be an infinite regression from one *buddhi*[76] to another, along with the confusion created by *smṛti*.

22. चितेरप्रतिसङ्क्रमयस्तदाकारपत्तौ स्वबुद्धिसंवेदनम्।

citeḥ-aprati saṅkramayaḥ-tadākārapattau sva-buddhi-saṁvedanam ।

The *citi*, which does not unite (with objects), becomes conscious of its *buddhi*, when (the *citta* gains) *tadākāratā*[77] with it.

23. द्रष्टृदृश्योपरक्तं चित्तं सर्वार्थम्।

draṣṭṛ-dṛśya-uparaktaṁ cittaṁ sarvārtham ।

A *citta* affected by the seer as well as the object of sight gains knowledge of all intended objects.

KAIVALYA AS THE ULTIMATE REALISATION OF PURUṢA (IV.24-34)

24. तदसङ्ख्येयवासनाभिश्चित्रमपि परार्थं संहत्यकारित्वात्।

tad-asaṁkhyeya-vāsanābhiḥ-citram-api para-arthaṁ saṁhatyakāritvāt ।

---

76. *buddhi* = intelligence, the faculty of judgement; one of the three constituent parts of the *antaḥkaraṇa* along with *mana* and *citta*.

77. *tadākāratā* = the same form as another thing.

That (*citta*), although present in diverse forms because of (the countless) *vāsanā*-s, exists for the sake of another because it produces combinations.

25. **विशेषदर्शिन आत्मभावभावनाविनिवृत्ति।**

viśeṣa-darśina ātma-bhāva-bhāvanā-vinivṛtti ।

For one, who has this special sight, there is a cessation of thoughts about the states of the *ātmā*.

26. **तदाविवेकनिम्नं कैवल्यप्राग्भारं चित्तम्।**

tadā-viveka-nimnaṁ kaivalya-prāgbhāraṁ cittam ।

Then the *citta* is brought down towards *viveka*, onward to *kaivalya*.

27. **तच्छिद्रेषु प्रत्ययान्तराणि संस्कारेभ्यः।**

tat-chidreṣu pratyaya-antarāṇi saṁskārebhyaḥ ।

Through the gaps in this (*citta* enter) other ideas (coming) from the *saṁskāra*-s.

28. **हानमेषां क्लेशवदुक्तम्।**

hānam-eṣāṁ kleśa-vat-uktam ।

The escape from these (*saṁskāra*-s) is like that which has been said for the *kleśa*-s.

29. **प्रसङ्ख्यानेऽप्यकुसीदस्य सर्वथा विवेकख्यातेर्धर्ममेघः समाधिः।**

prasaṁkhyāne'pi-akusīdasya sarvathā vivekakhyāteḥ-dharma-meghaḥ samādhiḥ ।

One, who is not miserly even after *prasaṁkhyāna*, always attains as a result of *viveka-khyāti*, a *samādhi* called *dharma-megha*.[78]

---

78. *dharma-megha* = (lit.) cloud of *dharma*; for *dharma* see Note 56 on III.13 probably refers to the whole range of *dharma*-s of an object that get visible to the seer on attainment of this *samādhi*.

prasaṁkhyāna = elevation.

30. ततः क्लेशकर्मनिवृत्ति

tataḥ kleśa-karma-nivṛtti ।

Thereafter (comes) the cessation of *kleśa* and *karma*.

31. तदा सर्वावरणमलापेतस्य ज्ञानस्यानन्त्याज्ज्ञेयमल्पम्

tadā sarva-āvaraṇa-mala-apetasya jñānasya-anantyāt-jñeyam-alpam ।

Then, all obscuring covers and impurities having been removed (from knowledge), because of the infinite nature of knowledge, what is yet to be known is little.

32. ततः कृतार्थानां परिणामक्रमसमाप्तिर्गुणानाम्।

tataḥ kṛtārthānāṁ pariṇāma-krama-samāptiḥ-guṇānām ।

When, as a result of this, the *guṇa*-s fulfil their purpose, the end to the sequence of *pariṇāma*-s is attained.

33. क्षणप्रतियोगी परिणामापरान्तनिर्ग्राह्यः क्रमः।

kṣaṇa-pratiyogī pariṇāma-aparānta-nirgrāhyaḥ kramaḥ ।

Sequence, as a counter to momentariness, becomes *grāhya* at the end of *pariṇāma*-s.

34. पुरुषार्थशून्यानां गुणानां प्रतिप्रसवः कैवल्यं स्वरूपप्रतिष्ठा वा चितिशक्तेरिति।

puruṣa-artha-śūṇyānāṁ guṇānāṁ pratiprasavaḥ kaivalyaṁ svarūpa-pratiṣṭhā vā citi-śakteḥ-iti ।

Kaivalya is the *pratiprasava* of *guṇa*-s, no longer provided with a purpose by the *puruṣa*, or it is the getting grounded in its *svarūpa* of the power of one's *citi*.

Appendix

Cognition and Signification in the Yoga System of Philosopy[1]

YOGA has acquired the status of almost a common noun in the English language and one tends to have some commonsensical ideas about its basic ethical precepts without really knowing what its philosophical universe is constitutive of. The focus in most popular treatises on Yoga is either on *haṭha-yoga* or the different physical exercises that have come to be associated with a practice of the philosophy, or on the highly mystical (and progressively more mystified) 'superhuman' powers that the Yoga system apparently provides the means to be a master of. This paper concentrates on neither and having realised the superficiality as well as the superfluity of such endeavours, proposes instead to look into how the primary text of the Yoga system of philosopy deals with the question of congnition and signification, and how its essential ethical prerogatives stem from these problematics themselves.

Yoga is one of the six *āstika* or orthodox[2] schools of classical

1. Published in *Language Forum*, Vol. 25, No. 2, 1999, and later in H.S. Gill and G. Manetti (eds.), *Signs and Signification*, Bahri, New Delhi: 2000.
2. The schools of Indian philosophy which believe in the supremacy of the Veda-s (viz. Mīmāṁsā, Nyāya, Sāṁkhya, Vedānta, Vaiśeṣika and Yoga) are called *āstika* or orthodox, while those which do not (viz. Cārvāka, Bauddha and Jaina) are called *nāstika* or heterodox. Being *āstika* has got nothing to do with believing in God, because among the six orthodox schools mentioned above, the first three are atheistic schools while the latter three believe in a concept called *īśvara*, roughly translatable as God.

Indian philosophy. In terms of its epistemology and ontology it relies heavily on the Sāṁkhya system, adding only one significant ontological category of *īśvara* (see note 1 on p. 63) to its elaborate system of twenty-five categories of reality. According to the Yoga-Sāṁkhya system, there are fundamentally two principles in reality: *puruṣa* or the primal self and *prakṛti* or primal matter, and though these two principles are essentially discrete, it is because of their assumed conjunction, brought about through different means, that this 'sorrowful' world of primarily erroneous perception or *māyā* is created. Yoga talks about how to get rid of 'sorrow' by dissociating these two fundamental principles and understanding the true nature of human cognition and signification.

The primary text of the Yoga system of philosophy is the *Yoga-sūtra* by Patañjali, and though it has been followed in traditional Yoga scholarship by eminent commentaries like the *Yoga-bhāṣya* by Vyāsa, the *Tattva-vaiśāradī* by Vācaspati, the *Yoga Maṇiprabhā* and the *Vitti* by Bhojarāja, and the *Yoga-vārttika* by Vijñānabhikṣu, I take up in this paper only the first text and make a close reading of its four books to bring out how the Yoga system analyses and explains the processes of human congnition and signification in a model markedly different from either of the two traditionally assumed dichotomous poles of materialism and idealism.

The *Yoga-sūtra*-s of Patañjali act more as a manual than a philosophical treatise and this is confirmed not only by the extremely aphoristic nature of its mnemonic rules but also by its very first *sūtra* — 'Now [follows an exposition of] the discipline of Yoga' (I.1)[3]. It is, however, this manual for a discipline that I wish to analyse to read from within it the Yoga conception of

3. All quotations from the text are my translations from the Sanskrit original. Apart from punctuations, articles, simple prepositions and the copula, extra words added either to give syntactical coherence to the aphorism or to explain its full sense have always been put in third brackets. The numbers given in first brackets at the end of each quotation indicates the volume and *sūtra* number.

cognition, language and representation. To do this, however, one needs to first understand the basic assumptions of the philosophical system.

Patañjali makes the first principle of his philosophy clear in the second *sūtra* itself: 'Yoga is the restriction of *vṛtti*-s of the *citta*' (I.2)[4]. For ancient Indian philosophy, the human cognising apparatus has three parts: the *manas*, or the immediate receptacle of knowledge, the *buddhi*, or the intellect that sieves the information thus gathered, and the *citta*, or the basal cognising apparatus which finally bears the imprints of the information to be retained. The imprints that knowledge leaves on the *citta* through various sources are called *vṛtti*-s, and therefore Yoga primarily talks about a restriction to regular modes of knowledge-formation itself. Having stated in the fifth *sūtra* that *vṛtti*-s can be of five types, the text cites them in *sūtra* I.6 as *pramāṇa* or valid epistemologies, *viparyaya* or false knowledge, *vikalpa* or linguistically constructed knowledge, *nidrā* or sleep, and *smṛti* or memory. That false knowledge, sleep and memory can lead to illusory forms of knowledge, which need to be restricted is commonsensical, but that Yoga gives a similar status to valid epistemologies and language too is significant. In I.7, Patañjali lists *pratyakṣa* or perception, *anumāna* or inference and *āgama* or testimonial knowledge as the valid epistemologies he is talking about and in the inclusion of all three of them in categories that have to be restricted, the text makes its diatribe against all conventional forms of knowledge clear. The *vṛtti* that is of more immediate concern to this paper is however *vikalpa*, which is defined as '*Vikalpa* is that which follows from the knowledge of words [alone] and does not refer to any [real or perceptible] object' (I.9), i.e., something like the

---

4. For many of the *sūtra*-s like this one I have chosen to retain a few Sanskrit terms in their original form to give them the status of technical terms and also avoid the unncessary ambiguities and imprecision that their English rendering could have led to. In all such cases, however, the discussion that accompanies the quotation explains the terms in English.

Witgensteinian 'horned tiger', which cannot exist in reality but can only be conceived as a linguistic construct. Language as an independent source of knowledge formation is thus as much negated in Yoga as is language as a secondary dispenser of information.

Having already stated that *vr̥tti*-s of the *citta* have to be restricted and having also identified the *vr̥tti*-s themselves, the text moves on next to talk about the means to do the same. In I.12, it mentions the first couple of means as *abhyāsa* or practice and *vairāgya* or the feeling of not being strongly attached towards something. 'Practice' is described as 'care taken towards making [the *citta*] stable there [i.e., in the restricted state] is *abhyāsa*' (I.13), but the second method of unattachedness or passionlessness is defined in more detail. The text says, '*Vairāgya* is the consciousness of one's control over the desire for seen or heard objects' (I.15), thereby connecting the principle of renunciatory control to one of the epistemologies — that of perception.

While this brings us to the problematics of knowledge and language in the domain of the means to restriction too, this association becomes clearer when Patañjali talks about the third means to restriction — 'Or [concentration leading to restriction of *vr̥tti*-s can be achieved] through contemplation on *īśvara*' (I.23)[5]. It had already been stated how the inclusion of *īśvara* as an ontological category marks Yoga as a philosophical system distinct from Sāṁkhya, but what is to be noted is that for Patañjali, *īśvara* is not really a deity but rather a special cognitive category. He characterises *īśvara* through three features. In *sūtra* I.24, he calls it a special type of *puruṣa* or self which is not affected by the latent deposits of *karma*[6]. In *sūtra*

---

5. I deliberately put *īśvara*, which is normally considered synonymous to 'God', in the small case to show how here it is not at all the unitary divine principle that is being talked about.

6. I do not explain *karma* within the main text of the paper because first, it is not a term of immediate technical consequence to this paper and secondly, because this word has almost acquired the status →

I.25, he identifies it with the seed of omniscience. Finally, as a third feature, he describes the category as 'The teacher of even the ancient ones [i.e., the sages] that which is not limited by time' (I.25). It can be observed from these three features that for Yoga ontology, the status of divinity is accorded to a cognitive category, a self that deals with knowing and teaching, rather than an omnipotent deity. This relationship between *īśvara* and knowledge and language is made clearer in the next *sūtra*, which says 'Its [i.e., *īśvara*'s] verbal form is the *praṇava* [i.e., the syllable *auṁ*[7]]' (I.27), and *sūtra* I.28 suggests that one should repeatedly utter this syllable and contemplate on its possible meaning. The category of *īśvara* thus becomes not just a cognitive entity but also a linguistic item.

The relationship between restriction of *vṛtti*-s and vocalisation is carried forward further in the fourth means of a controlled retention and letting out of breath that the text suggests in *sūtra* I.34. The next two means towards restriction — that of making the *citta* disinterested towards objects (I.37) and that of gaining insight from oneiric knowledge (I.38) — are relatively repetitive, but the final means suggested: 'Or through concentration on whatever one wishes' (I.39) shows the flexibility of this apparently rigid manual philosophical system.

All these means towards restricting *vṛtti*-s of the *citta* point towards one thing — that of a focussed concentration of the mind — which is referred to as *samādhi*, or a state of trance deliberately attained through concentration. At this point, one should notice how Patañjali provides a typology of the different types of *samādhi* attainable. There can be a type of Yoga which is *samprajñāta* or conscious of linguistic construction about

→ of a common noun in English. In any case, the word refers to one of the basic concepts of the classical Indian version of metempsychosis, which talks about the deeds of one's previous births forming latent deposits that determine the nature and destiny of one's future births.

7. This untranslatable concept is related to the idea of the supreme self being akin to sound (*śabdabrahman*), and this sound being humanly appropriable through the syllable *auṁ*, to articulate which one requires the involvement of all the parts of one's vocal apparatus.

objects, and another which is *asamprajñāta* or not conscious of these. Talking about the means through which the former is attainable, Patañjali says, '*Samprajñāta* [*samādhi* is attainable] through *vitarka* [i.e., debate and deliberation on 'coarse' objects], *vicāra* [i.e., contemplation on 'subtile'], objects [mental] happiness and the sense of selfhood' (I.17)[8]. Defining the type of *samādhi* not conscious of objects, the text says, 'The other type [of *samādhi*, i.e., the *asamprajñāta* one] is preceded by *abhyāsa* [i.e., practice as explained above], causes a cessation [of *vṛtti*-s] and ends with [nothing but] *saṁskāra*-s' (I.18). *Saṁskāra*-s are the impressions that *vṛtti*-s leave on one's mind and which go on to form one's set of convictions and beliefs and, in the final analysis, one's self, and one can appreciate that since *asamprajñāta* Yoga is not conscious of objects and it leads to a restriction of *vṛtti*-s in any case, the *saṁskāra* that is the end-product of this type of *samādhi* is of a different order from the normal *saṁskāra*-s. Terming the final stage of a *samādhi* as *samāpatti* or 'closure' (I.41), the text shows how depending on the two forms of *samādhi*, the final outcome might be of four types. What is interesting is that the distinction that Yoga philosophy draws at this stage is based solely on linguistic grounds. The first type is the one that arises out of the *samprajñāta* path of debate or deliberation on 'coarse' objects, i.e., *savitarkā samāpatti*: one that uses language and thus is limited within the linguistic constructions of *vikalpa*. The text says, 'Of these [different types of *samāpatti*], the *savitarkā samāpatti* is limited [and confused] by the *vikalpa*-ic triad of word, intended objects and idea' (I.42). The second type of *samāpatti* is the result of an *asamprajñāta* exercise on coarse objects, where, however, linguistic deliberation is not used and the *nirvitarkā samāpatti* can make cognition of objects possible without the mediation of language. For Patañjali, 'When memory

8. Though both *vitarka* and *vicāra* are easily translatable (I provide the translations immediately after the terms), I retain the Sanskrit original in the text because soon these two terms will be used in derivative forms (*savitarka* / *nirvitarka* and *savicāra* / *nirvicāra*) as technical terms.

is purified and [thoughts] emptied of their forms, bring out to light only the intended meaning, [it is] *nirvitarkā*' (I.43). The other two forms concern the 'subtile' objects and depending on whether it is *samprajñāta* or *asamprajñāta*, i.e., whether *vicāra*, or contemplation, has been used or not, they can be *savicārā* or *nirvicārā*, based again on the linguistic relation they entail. The text simply states, 'In a similar way [i.e., as was the case with *vitarka*], for subtile objects the *savicārā* and *nirvicārā* [*samāpatti*-s] get explained' (I.44). The text further goes on to say in I.45 that the *samāpatti* on these subtile objects terminates in what is *aliṅga*,[9] or what is the primary matter which does not have any differentiating markers associated to it. The text states in I.46 that these four types of *samāpatti*-s constitute the *sabīja samādhi* or the *samādhi* which has seeds attached to it, that is one that can lead on to newer *vṛtti*-s. However, out of these, the *nirvicārā* one is the most effective because the text says that, 'On mastering the *nirvicārā*, [one gets] internal calmness of the self' (I.47). The sepcial status of this type of *samāpatti* also results from the fact that '[This type of *samāpatti* has as its object] something different from the insight arising from heard or inferred objects, [because its object] arises from the [knowledge of the] particular intended object' (I.49). This speciality of this kind of *samādhi* results in the fact, as I.50 states that the *saṁskāra* produced out of this hinders the generation of any other *saṁskāra*. Thus, at the end of *nirvicāra*[10] *samādhi*, only one *saṁskāra* exists and if one can restrict that too, one can get rid of all *vṛtti*-s of the *citta*. This is the ultimate form of *samādhi*, the final goal of Yoga, the *nirbīja* or 'seedless' *samādhi*, and the

9. The term *aliṅga* literally means 'without *liṅga*', *liṅga* being the term for the differentiating markers used in language, especially that of gender. The term therefore refers to any concept that is undifferentiated.

10. So far, I had been using the term *nirvicārā*, i.e., with a terminal feminine marker *ā* because *samāpati* is a word in the feminine gender. Here, however, the word being used as an adjective for *samādhi*, which is masculine, the masculine form of the word — *nirvicāra* — is used.

first book concludes saying, 'On restricting even this [i.e., the last *saṁskāra* produced] everything is restricted [and there is] *nirbīja samādhi*' (I.51). Thus, that the Yoga system talks about *samādhi* as its primary agenda, but in laying out what this concept consists of, it presents an elaborate typology on the basis of its linguistic involvement and also presents an implicit hierarchy among these different forms of *samādhi*, which I wish to demonstrate in the figure below.

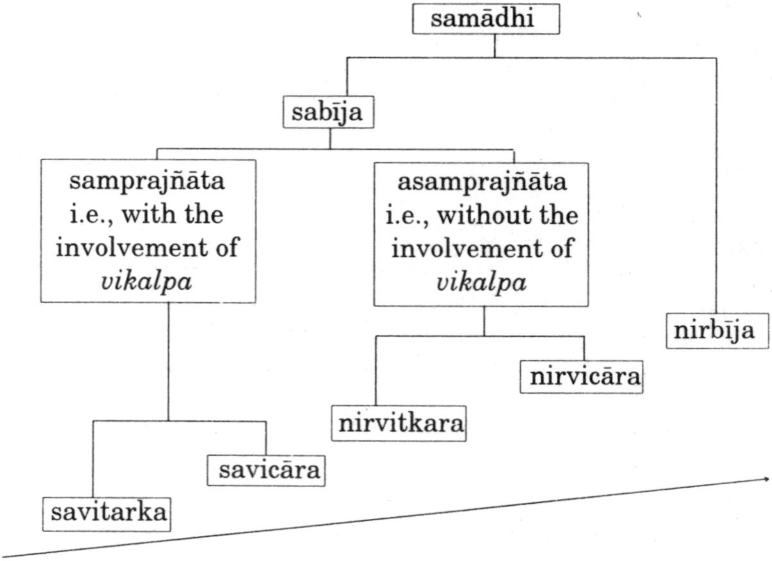

Figure 1. Different types of *samādhi* according to the Yoga system of philosophy. The arrow below the figure indicates the hierarchy entailed in the typology, whereby the lesser the involvement of language and cognition, the higher the status of that kind of *samādhi*.

After having stated the purpose and the different stages of Yoga in the first book of the *Yoga-sūtra*, Patañjali proceeds in the second book to lay down the means to achieve the ultimate stage of *nirbīja samādhi*. Before doing so, however, he adds that 'what is to be escaped [through Yoga] is sorrow which is yet to come' (II.16), to underline how the purpose of Yoga is basically to escape sorrow. The diatribe that Yoga launches against linguistic constructions and ordinary cognition in general is primarily because of the fact that language and normal cognition both operate on the basis of association, and it is the idea of association or *saṁyoga* between the self and matter or *puruṣa* and *prakṛti* that is for Yoga the root of all sorrow. Patañjali says, 'The cause behind what is to escaped [i.e., sorrow] is the association between the seer[11] and the object of sight' (II.17). In II.20 he states that the seer is nothing but the pure power of seeing, and in II.21 he shows how the phenomenalised object of sight exists only for the seer. Having shown how the seer or perceiver and the object perceived belong to two different levels of agency, Patañjali states in II.24 that in spite of this there is a tendency to imagine a one-to-one association between the two because of lack of proper knowledge (*avidyā*). If one can bring an end to this state of lack of proper knowledge, the sense of association that impedes the individual automatically stands escaped, and in the escape from this association with objects, the self attains the final stage of Yoga, that of *kaivalya* or isolation. The text says 'From the non-existence of this [i.e., of *avidyā* or lack of proper knowledge], association [between the self and objects] itself ceases to exist, and this is the escape, whereby the seer gains *kaivalya*' (II.25). The means to *kaivalya* thus lies in being able to discern and discriminate between the self and objects that surround the self, and in II.26, it is stated that the means to escape is unwavering *viveka-khyāti*[12] or the faculty of discriminative discernment. And this *viveka-khyāti* can be attained, as II.28 says through a practice of the different *aṅga*-s or the aids of Yoga.

Sūtra II.29 lists the eight *aṅga*-s of Yoga as *yama* or certain abstentions to be followed, *niyama* or certain observances to be made, *āsana* or certain postures of exercise, *prāṇāyāma* or a certain regulated control of breathing, *pratyāhāra* or a

---

11. Here 'seer' is not being used in the sense of a sage but as simply the person who sees. The Sanskrit word used in the text is *draṣṭā*.
12. The term *viveka*, refers to 'conscience' or the internal faculty of discerning, *khyāti* refers to the act of discrimination.

withdrawal of the senses, *dhāraṇā* or fixed attention, *dhyāna* or contemplative concentration, and *samādhi*. The first *aṅga* — that of abstention — is elaborated in II.30 as abstinence from violence, falsehood, theft, sexual excesses and receipt of material gifts. II.32 lists the types of observances to be made as the second *aṅga* of Yoga as cleanliness, contentment, self-castigation, self-study and contemplation on *īśvara*. The third aid of Yoga is defined as 'A stable [posture that produces] ease is *āsana*' (II.46). The second book of the text defines similarly the next two *aṅga*-s of *prāṇāyāma* and *pratyāhāra* in *sūtra*-s II.49 and II.54 respectively.

The remaining three *aṅga*-s are described separately in the third book of *Yoga-sūtra*, because as *sūtra* III.7 says these latter three *aṅga*-s are 'direct' aids of Yoga as compared to the first five which are more indirect in nature. The third book begins with a definition of these three direct *aṅga*-s. The sixth *aṅga* of fixed attention is defined as: 'Binding the *citta* to a fixed place is *dhāraṇā*' (III.1). *Sūtra* III.2 defines *dhyāna* as the singular focusing on the idea that arises out of *dhāraṇā*. The final *aṅga* of *samādhi*, which has been described earlier in the text in detail, is redefined here as 'Then [i.e., after *dhyāna*] when only the intended object gets illuminated, and it is moreover made free from its self, it is *samādhi*' (III.3). The text goes on to say in III.4 that these three direct *aṅga*-s together comprise *saṁyama* or constraint, and it is through different acts of *saṁyama* on different objects that the *yogī* or the individual practising Yoga can attain different powers.

After this, the text moves on to list the different things on which *saṁyama* can be practised and what powers can arise from these acts of constraint. While several rather esoteric powers, like how to vanish (III.21), how to penetrate another person's body (III.38) or how to float in the air (III.42) are listed in this stage of the text, I will focus only on those powers that immediately concern control over cognition and language. While it has earlier been shown how the basic principle of Yoga is to free oneself from linguistic constructions and commonplace cognition because of the principle of association involved therein, it has also been shown how Yoga does not preach an avoidance of knowledge *per se*, because the very working principle for its ultimate goal of *kaivalya* is the replacement of the usual *avidyā* or lack of knowledge with the true knowledge of isolation. Therefore, it is hardly surprising that among the different powers that a *yogī* can attain many are devoted to acquiring cognitive and linguistic skills.

The first power in this relation concerns the true understanding of linguistic signs. The text says, 'The word, the intended object and the idea are confusedly identified with each other [thereby leading to non-cognition in language and the resultant status of linguistic constructions in Yoga philosophy]. From a *saṁyama* on the differences among the three [arises] the knowledge of all worldly sounds'[13] (III.17). It is the knowledge of discernment that becomes thus of greatest importance and the text says, 'From a *saṁyama* on moments and their sequence [arises] knowledge of the *viveka* [i.e., discerning knowledge]' (III.52). Talking of discerning between what appears to be erroneously associated, the text goes on to show how *bhoga* or worldly experience itself arises from a confused identity between *sattva* or the immediately phenomenal self and *puruṣa* or the primal self and a true knowledge of the *puruṣa* arises from a dissociation of the two, by taking the sense of selfhood away from the *sattva*. It says, 'The experience of *bhoga* is the incapability to separate *sattva* and *puruṣa* which are [actually] very much unrelated. Since [the *sattva* is] the intended object of another [i.e., of the knowing self], from a *saṁyama* of [what exists for] its own sake arises the knowledge of the *puruṣa*' (III.35). Connecting this knowledge of the self with a mastery over the empirical means of perception, III.36 shows how this

13. The original term, which I have translated as 'knowledge of all worldly sounds', is *sarvabhūtarutajñānam*, which would literally mean 'knowledge of the cries of all worldly beings'. I have deliberately taken away the poetic element of the term without compromising on its basic sense.

saṁyama and the resultant knowledge of the *puruṣa* leads to the clarity of one's sense-organs. The text goes on to show in III.49 how one who has been able to dissociate the *sattva* from the *puruṣa* and thereby attained superior perceptive means comes to gain all knowledge. This is how the Yoga system talks about unlearning it all to finally gain true dissociative knowledge about all things. However, the isolationist culmination of Yoga in *kaivalya* requires, as it is stated in III.50, a disinterestedness in this acquired omniscience too, and *kaivalya* involves not just a dissociation of the self from matter but an isolation of the self from the very knowledge of this dissociation too.

The whole intention behind attaining *kaivalya* is to gain *siddhi* or perfection, and the fourth book of the text probes into the means to achieve this perfection. It begins by stating, 'States of perfection arises from birth, drugs,[14] *mantra*-s [i.e., incantatory spells], self-castigation and *samādhi*' (IV.1), and makes it clear in IV.6 that out of these means, that of *samādhi* is the best. Since what stands immediately in the way of attaining this *siddhi* is one's *vāsanā*-s or desires, the text moves on next to analyse what the causes behind desires are and what their nature is. *Sūtra* IV.8 says that desires are the expression of the fruition of one's *karma*, and IV.9 shows how, in spite of the roots of these desires being quite disjunct in time and space, one desire is causally related to another, because of the conjunction established by one's memory and the deposits of *saṁskāra*. Thus, the problematic category of desire is associated to the notion of causality as entailed in the functioning of the cognising apparatus, and IV.11 thus suggests that if one can remove the

---

14. That birth is a means to perfection comes from the classical Indian belief in *karma* or that one's destiny is determined to a great extent by the latent deposits from one's previous births, and are operative in an individual right from the onset of his or her current life. That drugs are also associated with traditional Indian ascetic practice. Different types of narcotics with traditional Indian ascetic practice. Different types of narcotic materials are used ritually in several Hindu festivals and are used to a great extent by *sādhu*-s of certain sects to heighten their levels of consciousness.

basic dependence of cognition on the chain of cause and effect, one can also bring desires to an end. The direction of Yoga practice is thus towards a dwindling of one's desires and a resultant dissociation of the self from material objects. *Sūtra* IV.25 says how a person who is able to see this distinction ceases to think about his or her self and 'then the *citta* sets down to the [discerning task of the] *viveka* and moves towards *kaivalya*' (IV.26).

Thus, *kaivalya*, the final isolationist stage of Yoga, deals with the dissociation of oneself from desire towards material objects as also a dissociative attempt in the means to cognition of these obejcts. The cessation of desire can itself lead to a dissociation of the self from matter (the assumed identity between which impedes true cognition of either) and a dissociation of the word from the intended object and idea (the assumed identity amongst which makes normal linguistic communication bereft of meaning), and 'true' dissociative knowledge and signification can arise out of this isolation of oneself from desire. The text says, 'Then [i.e., after this *kaivalya* from desire has been achieved], all obscuring coverings [of knowledge] having been removed, out of the endlessness of knowledge little is left to be known' (IV.31). It is this omniscience and mastery over all cognition and signification that is the final goal of Yoga philosophy, and the text ends on this note of freeing oneself from all conventional means of signification and cognition to gain finally a control over the dissociative and discrete nature of reality.

This polemic of Yoga philosophy against desire for material objects as well as the reliance of the knowing self on its association with matter might lead one to believe that Yoga represents an idealist system for which the act of individual thinking rather than the object of thought itself has got absolute reality. However, not only has it been observed that one of the goals of Yoga is to make possible the cognition of the object itself as unimpeded by ideas and signs, a series of *sūtra*-s in the fourth book actually argue against and disprove the basic premises of idealism. It is with a discussion of these *sūtra*-s that I would like to end my paper showing how Yoga corresponds neither to the idealist nor to the materialist poles of dominantly dichotomous Western thought, but instead talks of a dissociationist method where knowledge rests in being able to isolate the ideal self and matter without privileging either over the other. Showing how matter and the cognising self are sufficiently distinct, and the nature of the material object does not depend on transcendental subjective cognition, Patañjali says, 'The material object remains the same though the *citta*-s vary [and therefore the two have] different paths [of articulation and existence]' (IV.15). Moreover, since the *citta* cannot be a judge of itself, if material objects were formed by a single ideal self, their existence could never be proved. Patañjali says, 'And material objects do not depend upon a single *citta*, because [then] that would be unprovable [and] then what would the status [of that material object] be?' (IV.16). Rather, as IV.17 says, knowledge appears when a material object affects a *citta*, or two discrete entities get conjoint, without either being the root cause behind the other. Undercutting the idealistic presupposition of the thinking subject being itself the master of its knowledge, the text says, 'It [i.e., an individual *citta*] does not enlighten itself [with knowledge], because it is an object of sight [i.e., knowledge]' (IV.19). Knowledge of objects is thus formed neither by the transcendental knowing subject (because it is itself an object of knowledge and as objects themselves have an independent existence), nor by the objects themselves (because they need to be cognised to become knowledge), but rather by a simultaneous action of both these separate units on the mind. The text says, '[The knowledge of] all intended objects [arises from] the *citta* being affected by [both] the seer and the object of sight' (IV.23). It is this simultaneous action by the two disjoint and discrete units of the cognising self and the cognised object that creates the erroneous perception of a conjunction or association between the two (which is further aggravated by a hierarchisation of this conjunction by establishing either matter or mind as necessarily consumptive of the other as it is in the dichotomy of idealism and materalism), and it is this erroneous assumption of association that grants an illusory status to traditional cognition and signification. And this is where the Yoga system of philosophy brings in its idea of dissociation and isolation as also the manual means to achieve the same to lead, not to a nihilistic denial of all knowledge and meaning, but an establishment of the true nature of cognition and signification by showing how the subject and object of cognition and signification are essentially separate and disjoint.

Glossary and Index[1]

abhiniveśa [will to live]: II.3 (35); II.9 (36); note 34 (35).

abhyāsa [regular practice]: I.12 (27); I.13 (27); I.18 (28); I.32 (31); note 8 (27).

akliṣṭa [without *kleśa*; that which is not hindered or does not cause hindrance]: I.5 (26); note 4 (26).

aliṅga [without *liṅga* or markers of differentiation]: I.45 (34); II.19 (39); note 29 (34).

ananta [without an end]: II.47 (44); note 51 (44).

anādi [without a beginning]: IV.10 (57); note 73 (57).

aniṣṭa [harm]: III.51 (55); note 70 (55).

anitya [that which is not *nitya*; mutable]: II.5 (36); note 35 (36).

antarāya [obstacle]: I.29 (30); I.30 (31); note 20 (30).

antardhāna [the act of vanishing or becoming indiscernible]: III.21 (49); note 57 (49).

anumāna [ideational inference]: I.7 (26); I.49 (34); note 6 (26).

aṅga [organ, part]: II.28 (40); note 46 (40).

---

1. This is an index of the Sanskrit technical terms retained in the translation. The entries are alphabetically arranged as per the English alphabet. Wherever diacritics have occurred, however, first the parent letter occurs, followed by the diacritical letters in order of their occurrence in the Sanskrit alphabet. For example, words starting with 's' precede those starting with 'ś', which in turn precede those starting with 'ṣ'. Each entry comprises the Sanskrit term, its English equivalent in third brackets, the *sūtra* numbers in which it originates, the note number in which it is explained, and the page number of each occurrence in parentheses.

aṇimā [the state of an *aṇu* or atom]: III.45 (53) note 67 (53).

apavarga [liberation or salvation]: II.18 (38); note 42 (38).

ariṣṭa [signs of death]: III.22 (49); note 58 (49).

asamprajñāta [not conscious of objects; a type of *yoga*]: I.12[2] (28); note 12 (28).

asmitā [ego, feeling of personality]: I.17 (28); II.3 (35); II.6 (36); III.47 (54); IV.4 (56); note 11 (28).

avasthā [current state or condition]: III.13 (47); note 56 (47).

avidyā [non-knowledge, lack of knowledge]: II.3 (35); II.4 (36); II.5 (36); II.24 (39); note 34 (35).

aviśeṣa [non-particular]: II.19 (39); note 43 (39).

āgama [verbal testimonial knowledge]: I.7 (26); note 6 (26).

ānanda [happiness]: I.17 (28); note 11 (28).

āsana [postures of exercise]: II.29 (40); II.46 (43); note 48 (41).

āśaya [latent deposits of *karma*]: I.24 (29); II.12 (37); IV.6 (57); note 17 (29).

ātma / *ā*[3] [self, or essence of an entity]: II.5 (36); IV.13 (58); IV.25 (60); note 35 (36).

ātmadarśana [realising one's own self]: II.41 (43); note 50 (43).

bala [strength, physical power]: III.23 (49); III.24 (49); III.46 (54); note 59 (49).

bhoga [experience and acquisition of one's *karma*]: II.13 (37); II.18 (38); III.35 (51); note 39 (37).

bhūta [matter]: II.18 (38); III.13 (47); III.44 (53); note 42 (38).

buddhi [the intermediate cognising apparatus; the faculty of judgment, which sieves through all the data received by the *mana* before

---

2. The term *asamprajñāta* does not occur in the text at all, but is hinted at in I.18, and since it is a very important concept in *yoga*, I have included it here in the index.

3. Here I make a single entry for two forms of the same word. The word *ātmā* refers to the noun 'self', while the word *ātmā* refers to the adjective 'self'.

sending it to the *citta*]: I.21 (59); IV.22 (60); note 76 (59).

citi [the intentional cognising agency]: IV.22 (60); IV.34 (62); note 75 (58).

citta [the basal cognising apparatus where the sieved data sent over by *mana* are stored as imprints of perception]: I.2 (25); I.30 (31); I.37 (32); II.54 (45); III.1 (45); III.9 (47); III.11 (47); III.12 (47); III.19 (49); III.34 (51); III.38 (52); IV.4 (56); IV.5 (56); IV.15 (58); IV.16 (59); IV.17 (59); IV.18 (59); IV.21 (59); IV.23 (60); IV.26 (60); note 2 (25).

darśana-śakti [the power by which one sees, one's visual capacity]: II.6 (36); note 36 (36).

dharma [intrinsic properties which retain the *sattva* or the 'thatness' of an entity]: III.13 (47); III.14 (48); III.45 (53); IV.12 (58); note 56 (47).

dharma-megha [lit. cloud of *dharma*-s; probably refers to the whole range of *dharma*-s that an entity bears]: IV.29 (61); note 78 (61).

dharmī [a substance which has *dharma*]: III.14 (48).[4]

dhāraṇā [formation of ideas]: II.29 (41); II.53 (45); III.1 (45); note 48 (41).

dhyāna [contemplation through concentration]: I.39 (32); II.11(37); II.29 (41); III.2 (45); IV.6 (57); note 24 (32).

doṣa [fault or defect]: III.50 (54); note 69 (54).

dṛk-śakti [the power of seeing, vision itself]: II.6 (36); note 36 (36).

duḥkha [pain, sorrow]: II.15 (37); II.16 (38); II.34 (42); note 40 (38).

dvandva [turmoil; here within one's self]: II.48 (44); note 52 (44).

dveṣa [hatred]: II.3 (35); II.8 (36); note 34 (35).

grahaṇa [lit. the act of taking; here the act of cognising]: I.41 (33); III.47 (54); note 26 (33).

grahitā [lit. the one who takes; here the one who cognises]: I.41 (33); note 26 (33).

---

4. The term *dharmī* has not been provided with a footnote in the translation because III.14 itself gives a detailed definition of the term.

grāhya [lit. that which is taken; here that which is cognised]: I.41 (33); III.21 (49); IV.33 (62); note 26 (33).

guṇa [qualities or properties]: I.16 (28); II.15 (38); II.19 (39); IV.13 (58); IV.32 (61); IV.43 (62); note 10 (28).

indriya [bodily organs of sense or action]: II.18 (38); II.41 (43); II.54 (45) II.55 (45); III.13 (47); III.47 (54); note 42 (38).

īśvara [God; but in *yoga* more of a special cognitive category]; I.23 (29); I.24 (29); II.1 (35); II.32 (41); II.45 (43); note 16 (29).

japa [repeated utterance in the form of an incantation]: I.28 (30); note 19 (30).

kaivalya [lit. isolation; here isolating oneself from the *vṛtti*-s, synonymous with *apavarga*]; II.25 (40); III.50 (54); III.55 (55); IV.26 (60); IV.34 (62); note 44 (39).

karma [one's doings in life, which have an impact on one's after-lives]: I.24 (29); II.12 (37); III.22 (49); IV.7 (57); IV.30 (61); note 17 (29).

khyāti [the act of discernment]: I.16 (28); II.5 (36); III.49 (54); note 10 (28).

kleśa [cause of hindrance]: I.24 (29); II.2 (35); II.3 (35); II.12 (37); IV.28 (61); IV.30 (61); note 4 (26).

kliṣṭa [with *kleśa*; that which is hindered or causes hindrance]: I.5 (26); note 4 (26).

kriyā-yoga [the *yoga* of action]: II.1 (35); note 32 (35).

kūrma-nāḍī [a tortoise-shaped tube just beneath the human laryngo-oesophagal tract]: III.31 (51); note 60 (51).

lakṣaṇa [manifest properties]: III.13 (47); III.53 (55); note 56 (47).

liṅgamātra [merely with *liṅga* or the markers of differentiation; merely differentiable]: II.19 (39); note 43 (39).

mahāvideha [the great discarnate one; i.e., ***brahman***[5]]: III.43 (53); note 66 (53).

---

5. For detailed discussion on *brahman*, see the prefactory essay, "Six Indian Philosophical Systems and Patañjali's Yoga-sūtras", pp. 11-12.

mahāvrata [a great course of conduct]: II.31 (41); note 49 (41).

mana [the initial cognising apparatus which receives perceptual data]: I.35 (32); II.53 (45); III.48 (54); note 23 (32).

mūrdhā-joyti [cranial radiance]: III.32 (51); note 61 (51).

nimitta [the effective cause, as opposed to *prakṛti*, which is the evolving cause]: IV.3 (56); note 72 (56).

nirbīja [without seeds for future propagation]: I.51 (35); III.8 (46); note 30 (34).

nirodha [restriction; control aimed towards restriction]: I.2 (25); I.4 (25); I.5 (26); I.12 (27); I.51 (35); III.9 (47); note 2 (25).

nirvicāra / ā[6] [without *vicāra*]: I.43 (33); I.47 (34); note 28 (33).

nirvitarka / ā [without *vitarka*]: I.43 (33); note 27 (33).

nitya [unchanging, eternal]: II.5 (36); IV.10 (57); note 35 (36).

niyama [observance]: II.29 (40); II.32 (41); note 48 (41).

pariṇāma [mutation, the outcome]: II.15 (37); III.9 (47); III.11 (47); III.12 (47); III.13 (47); III.15 (48); III.16 (48); IV.2 (56); IV.14 (58); IV.18 (59); IV.32 (61); IV.33 (62); note 40 (38).

pradhāna [lit. principal; refers to the principal cause; synonymous with *prakṛti*]: III.48 (54); note 68 (54).

prajñā [insight]: I.20 (29); I.48 (34); I.49 (34); II.27 (40); III.5 (46); note 15 (29).

prakṛti [primal matter]: I.19 (28); IV.2 (56); IV.3 (56); note 14 (28).

pramāṇa [valid epistemologies]: I.6 (26); IV.16 (59); note 5 (26).

praṇava [the mystical syllable *auṁ*]: I.27 (30); note 18 (30).

prasaṁkhyāna [elevation, sublimation]: IV.29 (61); note 78 (61).

pratibhā [inner radiance; talent]: III.33 (51); III.36 (52); note 62 (51).

pratiprasava [inverse propagation]: II.10 (37); IV.34 (62); note 38 (37).

---

6. Here, as also in the cases of *nirvitarka*, *savicāra* and *nirvicāra*, I provide one entry for both the gendered forms that the words occur in the text in, because the gender marker depends simply on the gender of the word which follows and has no impact on its basic meaning.

pratyakcetanā [introverted consciousness]: I.29 (30); note 21 (30).

pratyakṣa [empirical perception]: I.7 (26); note 6 (26).

pratyāhāra [withdrawal, here of the senses]: II.29 (40); II.54 (45); note 48 (41).

pravṛtti [propensities]: I.35 (32); IV.5 (56); note 23 (32).

prāṇāyāma [regulated control of breath]: II.29 (40); II.49 (44); note 48 (41).

puruṣa [the primal conscious agency]: I.16 (28); III.35 (51); III.49 (54); III.55 (55); IV.18 (59); IV.34 (62); note 10 (28).

rasa [essence]: II.9 (36); note 37 (36).

rāga [passion]: II.3 (35); II.7 (36); note 34 (35).

ṛtambharā [bearer of *ṛta* or the frozen moment where immutable truth reveals itself]: I.48 (34); note 31 (34).

sabīja [with seeds for future propagation]: I.46 (34); note 30 (34).

samādhi [intense concentration leading to trance]: I.20 (29); I.46 (34); I.51 (35); II.2 (35); II.29 (41); II.45 (43); III.3 (46); III.11 (47); III.37 (52); IV.1 (56); IV.29 (61); note 15 (29).

samāna [movement of bodily fluids between the heart and the navel]: III.40 (52); note 65 (52).

samāpatti [conclusion, the final stable stage]: I.42 (33), II.47 (44); III.42 (53); note 25 (33).

samprajñāta [conscious of objects; a type of *yoga*]: I.17 (28); note 11 (28).

saṁskāra [subliminal impressions that *vṛtti*-s leave on the *citta*]: I.18 (28); I.50 (34); II.15 (37); III.9 (47); III.10 (47); IV.9 (57); IV.27 (61); note 13 (28).

saṁyama [the act of restrictive control]: III.4 (46); III.16 (48); III.17 (48); III.21 (49); III.22 (49); III.26 (50); III.35 (51); III.41 (53); III.42 (53); III.44 (53); III.47 (54); III.52 (55); note 54 (46).

saṁyoga [conjunction]: II.17 (38); II.23 (39); II.25 (40); III.18 (48); note 41 (38).

sattva [lit. thatness; the phenomenal essence of an entity]: II.41 (43);

III.35 (51); III.49 (54); III.55 (55); note 50 (43).

savicāra / ā [with *vicāra*]: I.44 (33); note 28 (33).

savitarka / ā [with *vitarka*]: I.42 (33); note 27 (33).

siddha-darśana [vision of the state of *siddhi* or fulfilment]: III.32 (51); note 61 (51).

siddhi [fulfilment]: III.37 (52); IV.1 (56); note 61 (51).

smṛti [memory, or mindfulness[7]]: I.6 (26); I.11 (27); I.20 (29); I.43 (33); IV.9 (57); IV.21 (59); note 5 (26); note 15 (29).

sthūla [coarse, materially tangible]: III.44 (53); note 11 (28).

sūkṣma [subtle, intangible]: I.44 (33); I.45 (34) II.10 (37); II.50 (44); III.25 (50); III.44 (53); IV.13 (58); note 11 (28).

svarūpa [one's own essential form]: I.3 (25); I.43 (33); II.54 (45); III.3 (46); III.44 (53); III.47 (54); IV.12 (58); IV.34 (62); note 3 (25).

tadākāratā [a thing attaining the same form as another thing]: IV.22 (60); note 77 (60).

tapaḥ [self-castigation]: II.1 (35); II.32 (41); II.43 (43); IV.1 (56); note 33 (35).

tāpa [anxiety]: II.15 (37); note 40 (38).

udāna [movement of bodily fluids from throat upwards]: III.39 (52); note 64 (52).

upasarga [symptoms of obstacles]: III.37 (52); note 63 (52).

vairāgya [passionlessness, renunciation]: I.12 (27); I.15 (27); III.50 (54); note 8 (27);

vastu [thing, object]: IV.14 (58); IV.15 (58); IV.16 (59); IV.17 (59); note 75 (58).

vaśīkāra [the power to control and be the master of]: I.15 (27); I.40 (32); II.55 (45); note 9 (27).

vāsanā [desire]: IV.8 (57); IV.24 (60); note 71 (56).

---

7. The term *smṛti* is used in these two different senses in the text. As 'memory', as used in I.6, I.11, I.43, IV.9, and IV.21, it is negative, being a *vṛtti* to be restricted through *yoga*; but as 'mindfulness', as in I.20, it is positive and one of the means to *samprajñāta yoga*.

vicāra [reflection on subtle intangible objects]: I.17 (28); note 11 (28).

vikalpa [knowledge derived only from linguistic constructs]: I.6 (26); I.9 (26), I.42 (33); note 5 (26); see also note 7 (26).

vikṣepa [distraction]: I.30 (31); I.31 (31); note 22 (31).

viparyaya [misconception]: I.6 (26); I.8 (26); note 5 (26).

vipāka [the fruition of one's *karma*-s]: I.24 (29); II.13 (37); IV.8 (57); note 17 (29).

viśeṣa [particular]: II.19 (39); note 43 (39).

vitarka [debate on material objects]: I.17 (28); II.33 (41); II.34 (42); note 11 (28).

viveka [the discriminative faculty]: III.52 (55); III.54 (55); IV.26 (60); note 40 (38).

viveka-khyāti [*khyāti* with *viveka*; discriminative discernment]: II.26 (40); II.28 (40); IV.29 (61); note 45 (40).

vivekin [one who has *viveka*]: II.15 (38); note 40 (38).

vṛtti [fluctuations caused in one's cognising apparatus on cognition]: I.2 (25); I.41 (33); II.11 (37); II.15 (38); II.50 (44); III.43; (53); IV.18 (59); note 2 (25).

vyakta [in the phenomenalised form]: IV.13 (58); note 74 (58).

vyutthāna [uprising]: III.9 (47); III.37 (52); note 55 (47).

yama [abstention]: II.29 (40); II.30 (41); note 48 (41).

yoga I.1 (25); I.2 (25); II.28 (40)[8].

yogī [one who performs *yoga*]: IV.7 (57).

---

8. The terms *yoga* and *yogī* have not been provided with footnotes in the translation because *yoga* is the subject of the whole book and cannot be suitably explained in a footnote. One can read the 'Introduction', the 'Prefatory Essay' and the 'Appendix' to have some idea about the meaning of the word *yoga*.